T0292672

CASE REVIEW
Thoracic Imaging

Series Editor
David M. Yousem, MD, MBA
Director of Neuroradiology and Professor of Radiology
Johns Hopkins Hospital
Vice Chairman of Program Development
Russell H. Morgan Department of Radiology and Radiological Science
The Johns Hopkins Medical Institutions
Baltimore, Maryland

Other Volumes in the CASE REVIEW Series
Brain Imaging, Second Edition
Breast Imaging
Cardiac Imaging
Emergency Radiology
Gastrointestinal Imaging, Second Edition
General and Vascular Ultrasound
Genitourinary Imaging
Head and Neck Imaging, Third Edition
Musculoskeletal Imaging, Second Edition
Nuclear Medicine, Second Edition
Obstetric and Gynecologic Ultrasound, Second Edition
Pediatric Imaging
Spine Imaging
Vascular and Interventional Imaging

Phillip M. Boiselle, MD
Associate Professor of Radiology
Harvard Medical School;
Vice Chair of Quality, Safety and Performance
   Improvement
Director, Thoracic Imaging Section
Beth Israel Deaconess Medical Center
Boston, Massachusetts

Gerald F. Abbott, MD
Associate Professor of Diagnostic Imaging
Warren Alpert Medical School of Brown University
Providence, Rhode Island;
Associate Radiologist of Division of Thoracic Imaging
   and Intervention
Massachusetts General Hospital
Boston, Massachusetts

Theresa C. McLoud, MD
Professor of Radiology
Harvard Medical School;
Associate Radiologist-in-Chief
Director of Education
Thoracic Radiologist
Massachusetts General Hospital
Boston, Massachusetts

CASE REVIEW

Thoracic Imaging

SECOND EDITION

CASE REVIEW SERIES

ELSEVIER
MOSBY

1600 John F. Kennedy Blvd
Ste 1800
Philadelphia, PA 19103-2899

THORACIC IMAGING: CASE REVIEW, SECOND EDITION   ISBN: 978-0-323-02999-5

Notices

Knowledge and best practice in this field are constantly changing. As new research and experience broaden our understanding, changes in research methods, professional practices, or medical treatment may become necessary.

Practitioners and researchers must always rely on their own experience and knowledge in evaluating and using any information, methods, compounds, or experiments described herein. In using such information or methods they should be mindful of their own safety and the safety of others, including parties for whom they have a professional responsibility.

With respect to any drug or pharmaceutical products identified, readers are advised to check the most current information provided (i) on procedures featured or (ii) by the manufacturer of each product to be administered, to verify the recommended dose or formula, the method and duration of administration, and contraindications. It is the responsibility of practitioners, relying on their own experience and knowledge of their patients, to make diagnoses, to determine dosages and the best treatment for each individual patient, and to take all appropriate safety precautions.

To the fullest extent of the law, neither the Publisher nor the authors, contributors, or editors, assume any liability for any injury and/or damage to persons or property as a matter of products liability, negligence or otherwise, or from any use or operation of any methods, products, instructions, or ideas contained in the material herein.

Previous edition copyrighted 2001 by Mosby, Inc.

International Standard Book Number 978-0-323-02999-5

Acquisitions Editor: Rebecca Gaertner
Developmental Editor: David Mack
Publishing Services Manager: Pat Joiner-Myers
Project Manager: Marlene Weeks
Design Direction: Steve Stave

Printed in the United States of America

Last digit is the print number: 9 8 7 6 5 4 3 2 1

Working together to grow
libraries in developing countries

www.elsevier.com | www.bookaid.org | www.sabre.org

ELSEVIER BOOK AID International Sabre Foundation

To my wife, Ellen
PMB

To my brother, Terry
GFA

To my sister, Veronica
TCM

What is more fundamental to radiology than thoracic imaging? Radiology training no doubt starts here for most residents, and yet the depth of investigation into cardiopulmonary pathology stretches into the final year of residency (or fellowship) training. The lungs and heart yield ever greater challenges to the reader, even as our imaging modalities get more and more sophisticated … or perhaps because our imaging modalities get more and more sophisticated. So it is that the *Thoracic Imaging: Case Review,* second edition, grows and grows and deals with disease in an even more intelligent manner.

I am grateful to Drs. Boiselle, Abbott, and McLoud for their hard work in assembling a group of cases that span the gamut from basic pathology to complicated disease. In addition they have allowed my goal of taking the Series to the next higher plane, that of an on-line interactive tool, to be realized for chest pathology. I think that the print format has its many advantages, but the electronic format also offers unique ways to teach. The Case Review Series must be adaptable and change with the ways trainees think and study. The authors of *Thoracic Imaging* have embraced these concepts and have helped enormously in launching not only their second edition, but also the Case Review Series of the future.

I hope you enjoy *Thoracic Imaging,* second edition, whether you are currently reading hard copy or soft copy … or both. Great job, Doctors!

David M. Yousem, MD, MBA

The presentation and discussion of "unknown" cases is an integral component of formal diagnostic radiology education. The Case Review Series uses this established format as a means of providing focused, subspecialty examination preparation for radiology residents. This book, *Thoracic Imaging*, also serves as a practical review for fellows and practicing radiologists who wish to sharpen their skills in this area.

This second edition of *Thoracic Imaging* maintains the same two primary goals as the original edition. First, it uses a case format presentation to illustrate and review the imaging features of disorders that span the spectrum of thoracic diseases with which a graduating resident should have a working familiarity. Accordingly, *Thoracic Imaging* comprises a diverse group of more than 150 cases using images from several modalities, including conventional radiography, computed tomography, high-resolution computed tomography, magnetic resonance imaging, and positron emission tomography. Similar to other books in this series, the cases are categorized by level of difficulty: Opening Round, Fair Game, and Challenge. Each case is followed by a list of questions, with answers provided on the verso page. The answers are followed by a brief discussion section that emphasizes characteristic imaging features, differential diagnostic considerations, and key points of clinical information for each case. For readers who desire additional information about a given topic, we have included a helpful reference for further reading. A cross-reference to *Thoracic Radiology: THE REQUISITES* is also provided.

Second, it is our goal to help the reader develop a sound framework with which to approach image interpretation in thoracic radiology. As teachers of radiology, we place dual emphasis on methodology and final diagnosis, believing that the means by which one reaches the final diagnosis is as important as arriving at a correct answer. Indeed, for some of the cases in this book, a specific, correct diagnosis is not expected from the reader.

In preparing this second edition of *Thoracic Imaging*, we have carefully updated the text, references and selected images from the first edition. We have also added new case material to cover important recent advances in a variety of thoracic imaging topics, including subsolid lung nodules, smoking-related lung diseases, emerging infections, idiopathic interstitial pneumonias, and the Fleischner Society guidelines for management of pulmonary nodules, among others. The addition of this new material was spearheaded by Dr. Gerald F. Abbott, who brought a creative and fresh perspective to this work.

This book is a collaborative project that has benefitted from the help of many. We are especially grateful to: Rebecca Gaertner, our editor at Elsevier, for editorial assistance; Dr. David Yousem, the editor of this series, for support and guidance; and Nancy Williams, for administrative assistance.

We hope that this new edition of *Thoracic Imaging* will continue to prove a valuable learning tool for its readers.

Phillip M. Boiselle, MD
Gerald F. Abbott, MD
Theresa C. McLoud, MD

Opening Round

1. Which imaging feature of this nodule is of concern for malignancy?

2. Which cell type of lung cancer is most likely?

3. What are the size criteria for a T2a lesion in the recent revision of the TNM (tumor-node-metastases) staging system?

4. Is this lesion better suited to image-guided transthoracic needle biopsy or bronchoscopic biopsy?

Lung Cancer

1. Spiculated margins.

2. Adenocarcinoma.

3. >3 cm but ≤5 cm in greatest dimension.

4. Transthoracic needle biopsy.

Reference

Müller NL, Silva CIS: Nodules and masses. In: Silva CIS, Müller NL, Eds. *Imaging of the Chest.* Philadelphia, Saunders, 2008, pp 136-157.

Cross-Reference

Thoracic Radiology: THE REQUISITES, 2nd ed, pp 284-286.

Comment

A *solitary pulmonary nodule* is defined as a well-circumscribed round or oval lesion measuring less than 3 cm in diameter. There are only two specific and reliable signs of benignancy on chest radiographs: (1) identification of a benign pattern of calcification or (2) demonstration of absolute absence of growth over a 2-year period. For cases that do not meet one of these criteria, thin-section CT is generally recommended for further evaluation. In comparison with radiography, CT allows a more accurate assessment of the margins of a nodule; moreover, CT is more sensitive for identifying the presence and distribution of calcium and fat within a nodule.

The nodule in this case has spiculated margins, a finding that is highly suspicious for malignancy. Depending on local practice patterns and clinical circumstances, a preoperative biopsy may be requested. The peripheral location of this nodule makes it best suited for a transthoracic needle biopsy.

The most common cell type of lung cancer is adenocarcinoma. It most often presents as a solitary, peripheral nodule with spiculated margins. Based on size criteria outlined in recent revisions to the TNM staging system for lung cancer, this 4.0-cm mass is a T2a lesion. The revisions establish the following size cut-off points for T designations: T1a: tumor ≤2 cm in greatest dimension; T1b: tumor >2 cm but ≤3 cm in greatest dimension; T2a: tumor >3 cm but ≤5 cm in greatest dimension; T2b: tumor >5 cm but ≤7 cm in greatest dimension; T3: tumor >7 cm (see *Thoracic Radiology: THE REQUISITES*, Table 11-1).

Notes

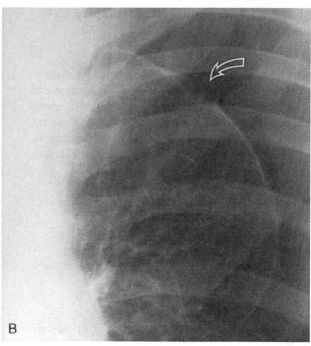

1. What is the cause of this patient's pleuritic chest pain and dyspnea?

2. Name at least five causes of pneumothorax.

3. Based on the imaging findings in this case, what is the most likely cause for this "spontaneous" pneumothorax?

4. What radiographic finding(s) in this case suggests the possibility of a tension pneumothorax?

Spontaneous Pneumothorax Secondary to Ruptured Bleb

1. Pneumothorax.

2. Spontaneous, chronic obstructive pulmonary disease, chronic infiltrative lung disease (e.g., Langerhans cell histiocytosis and lymphangioleiomyomatosis), malignant neoplasms (e.g., metastatic sarcoma), trauma, catamenial pneumothorax, iatrogenic, barotrauma, and infection (e.g., lung abscess and septic infarcts).

3. Ruptured apical bleb.

4. Depression of the left hemidiaphragm; expansion of the left rib cage.

Reference

O'Connor AR, Morgan WE: Radiological review of pneumothorax. *BMJ* 330:1493-1497, 2005.

Cross-Reference

Thoracic Radiology: THE REQUISITES, 2nd ed, pp 386-389.

Comment

Pneumothorax is defined as the presence of air or gas within the pleural space. Although there are a wide variety of causes, spontaneous pneumothorax is the most common etiology. Affected patients are usually in the third or fourth decade of life.

Spontaneous pneumothoraces are almost always secondary to rupture of an apical bleb, which represents a gas pocket within the elastic fibers of the visceral pleura. Note the presence of a small bleb along the visceral pleural margin in this patient, best demonstrated on the coned-down image of the left upper lobe (*arrow*, second figure). Such blebs have been reported to be detectable on chest radiographs in approximately 15% of cases of spontaneous pneumothorax. However, blebs are rarely evident on chest radiographs following resolution of the pneumothorax. CT is much more sensitive than radiography for detecting blebs and has been shown to detect blebs in approximately 80% of patients following resolution of spontaneous pneumothoraces. The size and number of apical blebs detected on CT have been shown to correlate with the risk of recurrent pneumothoraces and the need for surgical intervention.

Tension pneumothorax is a life-threatening condition. Affected patients present with clinical signs of tachypnea, tachycardia, cyanosis, sweating, and hypotension. Radiographic findings may include contralateral mediastinal shift, diaphragmatic depression, rib cage expansion, and flattening of the contours of the right heart border and/or venae cavae.

Notes

1. Where is this central venous catheter located?

2. Should the catheter be repositioned?

3. What is the most common complication of inadvertent placement of a catheter in this location?

4. Is inadvertent azygos vein cannulation more common following a left- or a right-sided vascular insertion approach?

Malpositioned Catheter in the Azygos Vein

1. Azygos vein.

2. Yes.

3. Venous rupture.

4. Left-sided.

Reference

Bankier AA, Reinhold M, Weismayr MN, et al: Azygos arch cannulation by central venous catheters: radiographic detection of malposition and subsequent complications. *J Thorac Imaging* 12:64-69, 1997.

Cross-Reference

Thoracic Radiology: THE REQUISITES, 2nd ed, pp 140-144.

Comment

Inadvertent insertion of a catheter into the azygos vein is a relatively uncommon complication of central venous catheter placement, with an estimated frequency of approximately 1%. Detection of a malpositioned catheter at this site is important, because there is a relatively high frequency of associated venous perforation.

Note the abnormal curve of the catheter at the level of the azygos arch on the posteroanterior (PA) chest radiograph. The precise location is confirmed on the lateral chest radiograph (second figure), which demonstrates the posterior course of the catheter within the azygos arch.

Interestingly, azygos vein cannulation occurs most commonly following left-sided catheter insertion. This association is thought to occur secondary to anterocaudal arching of the left brachiocephalic vein, which may preferentially promote entry of a catheter into the azygos vein rather than the superior vena cava. In contrast, catheters placed from the right side of the thorax have a more direct course to the superior vena cava via the right brachiocephalic vein.

Notes

1. Based on the imaging findings in this case, name several likely prior occupational settings for this individual.

2. Are pleural plaques from prior asbestos exposure usually unilateral or bilateral?

3. Are these lesions symptomatic?

4. Are pleural plaques premalignant?

C A S E 4

Calcified Pleural Plaques From Prior Asbestos Exposure

1. Mining, insulation manufacturing, textile manufacturing, construction, ship building, and brake lining manufacturing and repair.

2. Bilateral.

3. No.

4. No.

Reference

McLoud TC: Conventional radiography in the diagnosis of asbestos-related disease. *Radiol Clin North Am* 30:1177-1189, 1992.

Cross-Reference

Thoracic Radiology: THE REQUISITES, 2nd ed, pp 206-213.

Comment

The chest radiograph demonstrates numerous partially calcified lesions bilaterally, several of which are plateau-like in configuration and parallel the inner margin of the lateral thoracic wall and the right hemidiaphragm. CT confirms the pleural location of these lesions and demonstrates the calcification more precisely. The findings are typical of pleural plaques related to prior asbestos exposure.

Pleural plaques are the most common manifestation of asbestos exposure and typically occur after a latency period of approximately 15 to 20 years. They do not cause symptoms and are usually discovered incidentally. Pathologically, pleural plaques are composed of dense bands of avascular collagen and are not considered premalignant lesions.

The radiographic appearance of pleural plaques is dependent on whether the plaques are calcified, and whether they are seen in profile or *en face*. When observed in profile, a plaque appears as a dense band of soft tissue opacity paralleling the inner margin of the lateral thoracic wall or an adjacent hemidiaphragm. When observed en face, a plaque appears as a veil-like opacity with irregular edges, often described as a "holly leaf" configuration. Plaques are usually bilateral and often symmetric. The lower half of the thorax is most often affected, usually between the sixth and the ninth ribs.

Notes

1. Displacement of the paraspinal lines implies an abnormality in which mediastinal compartment?

2. Are thoracic vertebral body fractures commonly associated with mediastinal hematoma?

3. How reliable are portable chest radiographs and thoracolumbar radiographs for detecting spinal fractures?

4. Which portion of the spine is most susceptible to traumatic injury?

Vertebral Body Fracture With Paraspinal Hematoma

1. Posterior.

2. Yes.

3. Not very reliable.

4. The thoracolumbar junction (T12-L2).

Reference
Wintermark M, Mouhsine E, Theumann N, et al: Thoracolumbar spine fractures in patients who have sustained severe trauma: depiction with multi-detector row CT. *Radiology* 227:681-689, 2003.

Cross-Reference
Thoracic Radiology: THE REQUISITES, 2nd ed, pp 162, 165, 166, 375, 377.

Comment
Thoracic spine fracture is an infrequent but serious complication of blunt trauma. Unfortunately, the portable trauma chest radiograph is not very reliable in detecting spinal fractures. Moreover, thoracolumbar spine radiographs have been shown to have a sensitivity of only 32% for detecting acute spinal fractures.

Radiographic findings associated with spinal fracture include findings related to mediastinal hemorrhage (such as widening of the paraspinal lines, mediastinal widening, and left apical pleural cap) and vertebral abnormalities. The latter are more specific for spinal injury and include loss of height of the vertebral body and obscuration of the pedicle(s). When you identify a mediastinal hematoma that is confined to the posterior mediastinum, you should diligently search for evidence of a vertebral body fracture. If a spinal fracture is not evident on chest radiography, you should proceed to CT. Multidetector CT (MDCT) has been shown to have a much higher sensitivity than radiographs for detecting fractures and its sensitivity can be further enhanced by coronal and sagittal reformations.

Notes

A

B

1. What are the two major chest radiographic features of emphysema?

2. What is the best chest radiographic indicator of over-inflation of the lungs?

3. Is the chest radiograph a reliable tool for detecting emphysema?

4. What is the most sensitive imaging modality for detecting emphysema?

Emphysema

1. Overinflation of the lungs and reduced vascularity.

2. Flattening of the hemidiaphragms.

3. No.

4. High-resolution CT (HRCT) of the chest.

Reference

Webb WR: Radiology of obstructive pulmonary disease. *AJR Am J Roentgenol* 169:637-647, 1997.

Cross-Reference

Thoracic Radiology: THE REQUISITES, 2nd ed, pp 242-248.

Comment

Emphysema is defined as permanent, abnormal enlargement of airspaces distal to the terminal bronchiole, accompanied by destruction of their walls.

Radiographic abnormalities in patients with emphysema are related to overinflation of the lungs and lung destruction. The latter is characterized by reduced vascularity or the presence of bullae. Overinflation of the lungs may be characterized by a number of findings, most notably flattening of the hemidiaphragms and an increase in the retrosternal airspace diameter.

Chest radiographic abnormalities are usually evident in moderate to severe cases of emphysema, but radiographs are frequently normal in patients with early emphysema. HRCT is superior to chest radiographs in detecting and characterizing emphysema and has a high sensitivity and specificity for establishing the diagnosis.

Notes

1. What infection is most commonly associated with this pattern?

2. In cases of miliary tuberculosis (TB), how is the infection disseminated to the lung?

3. What other type of infection commonly presents with a miliary pattern?

4. Name four noninfectious entities that may present with a miliary pattern.

Miliary Tuberculosis

1. Miliary TB.

2. Hematogenously.

3. Fungal infection.

4. Pneumoconioses (e.g., silicosis), Langerhans cell histiocytosis, sarcoidosis, and metastases (e.g., thyroid, melanoma).

Reference

Reed JC: Diffuse fine nodular opacities. In: *Chest Radiology: Plain Film Patterns and Differential Diagnoses*, fifth edition. Philadelphia, Mosby, 2003, pp 287-303.

Cross-Reference

Thoracic Radiology: THE REQUISITES, 2nd ed, pp 104, 105.

Comment

A *miliary pattern* refers to the presence of numerous small (approximately 1- to 2-mm-diameter) lung nodules. Such nodules are difficult to detect radiographically because of their small size. It has been suggested that these tiny nodules become visible radiographically because of the effect of summation.

The classic entity associated with this pattern is miliary TB, which refers to the diffuse hematogenous dissemination of TB. This pattern typically occurs in patients with altered host resistance to the primary infection. Affected patients usually present with fever, chills, and night sweats.

Because of the small size of miliary nodules, it is not surprising that CT (particularly HRCT) is more sensitive than radiography for detection. In fact, it has been estimated that it may take up to 6 weeks for miliary nodules to become apparent on chest radiographs! On HRCT, the nodules are shown to be diffuse and random in distribution.

Notes

1. Where are the nodular opacities located?

2. What imaging feature on the PA radiograph suggests this location?

3. What is the most common chest wall structure to appear as a nodular opacity on a chest radiograph?

4. How can you confirm a suspected cutaneous site of a nodular opacity using chest radiography?

Neurofibromas

1. Chest wall.

2. Incomplete, sharp borders.

3. The nipples.

4. Repeat the radiograph with a small lead marker on the site of the cutaneous abnormality.

Reference

Reed JC: Chest wall lesions. In: *Chest Radiology: Plain Film Patterns and Differential Diagnoses*, fifth edition. Philadelphia, Mosby, 2003, pp 6-24.

Cross-Reference

Thoracic Radiology: THE REQUISITES, 2nd ed, pp 40-41.

Comment

When visible on chest radiographs, cutaneous chest wall lesions such as neurofibromas, moles, and nipples demonstrate a characteristic incomplete, sharp border. The sharp border is produced by the interface of the lesion with adjacent air, and it becomes incomplete where the lesion is continuous with the soft tissues of the chest wall. The identification of such a border is helpful for differentiating chest wall lesions from intrapulmonary lesions.

In this particular case, the cutaneous location of the nodules is easily confirmed on the lateral projection. When in doubt about a possible cutaneous location of a focal nodular opacity, one should perform a repeat radiograph with small lead markers for confirmation.

Notes

1. What is the diagnosis?

2. Name two primary signs of atelectasis.

3. Name five secondary signs of atelectasis.

4. What is the most common mechanism for complete lobar collapse?

C A S E 9

Complete Left Lower Lobe Atelectasis

1. Complete left lower lobe atelectasis.

2. Opacification of the affected lobe and displacement of the interlobar fissures.

3. Elevation of the hemidiaphragm, mediastinal shift, displacement of the hilum, compensatory hyperinflation, and crowded vessels.

4. Obstruction of a central bronchus.

Reference

Woodring JH, Reed JC: Radiographic manifestations of lobar atelectasis. *J Thorac Imaging* 11:109-144, 1996.

Cross-Reference

Thoracic Radiology: THE REQUISITES, 2nd ed, pp 31-40.

Comment

Atelectasis is defined as a decrease in volume (i.e., reduced inflation) of all or a portion of the lung. The most common type of atelectasis occurs secondary to obstruction of a central bronchus. It is referred to as *resorption atelectasis* and usually involves an entire lobe.

The chest radiograph and CT image reveal the classic features of complete left lower lobe atelectasis. On chest radiographs, complete left lower lobe atelectasis appears as a triangular opacity behind the heart. The displaced major fissure is seen as an interface between the opacified atelectatic lobe and the hyperexpanded left upper lobe. Note the presence of several secondary signs of atelectasis in this case, including inferomedial displacement of the left hilum, slight leftward shift of the mediastinum, and compensatory hyperinflation of the left upper lobe.

In an outpatient setting, the presence of lobar collapse is usually indicative of an obstructing central mass. In an adult patient, primary lung cancer and carcinoid are important diagnostic considerations. In a child, an aspirated foreign body is the most likely diagnosis. CT is helpful in identifying the centrally obstructing lesion and for guiding bronchoscopic procedures.

Notes

1. What disorder of pulmonary vascularity is evident in this case?

2. What is the difference between primary and secondary pulmonary artery hypertension (PAH)?

3. Is primary PAH more common in men or women?

4. Does a normal chest radiograph exclude the diagnosis of PAH?

CASE 10

Primary Pulmonary Artery Hypertension

1. PAH.

2. In secondary PAH, the hypertension has a known cause; in primary PAH, the cause is unknown.

3. Women.

4. No.

Reference

Frazier AA, Galvin JR, Franks TJ, Rosado-de-Christenson, M: From the Archives of the AFIP: Pulmonary vasculature: hypertension and infarction. *Radiographics* 20:491-524, 2000.

Cross-Reference

Thoracic Radiology: THE REQUISITES, 2nd ed, pp 327-330.

Comment

PAH is defined as a condition of sustained elevation of pulmonary artery pressure. PAH may occur secondary to one of three basic mechanisms: (1) increased pulmonary blood flow (e.g., left-to-right shunt), (2) decreased cross-sectional area of the pulmonary vasculature (e.g., chronic pulmonary embolism), and (3) increased resistance to pulmonary venous drainage (e.g., mitral valve disease). Another framework for categorizing causes of PAH is to broadly divide them as either precapillary (changes limited to the arterial pulmonary circulation) or post-capillary (primary abnormalities within the pulmonary venous circulation).

The majority of cases of PAH occur secondary to a known cause. These cases are collectively referred to as *secondary PAH.* In a minority of cases, the etiology of PAH remains unknown. These cases are referred to as *primary PAH.* This condition tends to affect women younger than 40 years of age.

Regardless of the type of PAH, the characteristic findings on chest radiographs are similar. There is usually marked enlargement of the main and hilar pulmonary arteries, which rapidly taper as they course distally. The degree of pulmonary artery enlargement varies considerably, and significant PAH can be present in the setting of a normal chest radiograph. CT is more accurate than chest radiography for detecting pulmonary artery enlargement.

Notes

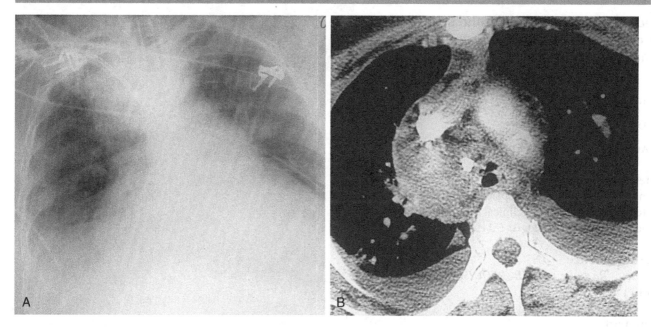

1. What is the most likely cause of mediastinal hematoma in this patient?

2. What is the most common complication of central catheter placement?

3. What is the optimal location for a central venous catheter?

4. Name two complications associated with catheter placement in the right atrium.

CASE 11

Mediastinal Hematoma Secondary to Vascular Perforation by a Central Venous Catheter

1. Vascular perforation by central venous catheter.

2. Malposition.

3. The superior vena cava.

4. Arrhythmia and cardiac perforation.

Reference
Kidney DD, Deutsch LS: Misplaced central venous catheters: venous anatomy, clinical significance, and treatment options. *Radiologist* 5:119-126, 1998.

Cross-Reference
Thoracic Radiology: THE REQUISITES, 2nd ed, pp 140-144.

Comment
Published rates of complications of central venous catheter placement vary considerably and are dependent upon both operator experience and anatomic site. The most common complication of central venous catheter placement is malposition, which occurs in up to 40% of cases. Pneumothorax is the second most common complication, occurring in up to 5% of cases. Less common complications include hemothorax, extrapleural hematoma, cardiac arrhythmias, vascular or cardiac perforation, peripheral venous thrombosis, catheter fragmentation, septic emboli, and mycotic aneurysms.

Because of its high flow rate and large volume, the superior vena cava is the ideal location for a central venous catheter. The distal portion of the catheter should lie parallel to the direction of blood flow, and it should not abut the vessel wall.

Catheter malposition is usually evident on a frontal chest radiograph. In some cases, however, a lateral view is necessary to determine the precise location of the catheter tip. In a small minority of cases, a contrast study is necessary to verify catheter location.

In this case, note the unusual medial course of the catheter on the chest radiograph. The CT image confirms an extravascular location.

Notes

1. What is the most common cause of bilateral, symmetric hilar lymph node enlargement?

2. What percentage of sarcoid patients with hilar lymphadenopathy also have lung parenchymal disease on chest radiography?

3. What percentage of patients with sarcoidosis are asymptomatic at the initial presentation?

4. Are noncaseating granulomas specific for sarcoidosis?

Sarcoidosis

1. Sarcoidosis.

2. Approximately 50%. May be higher on CT.

3. Approximately 50%.

4. No.

Reference

Miller BH, Rosado-de-Christenson ML, McAdams HP, Fishback NF: Thoracic sarcoidosis: radiologic-pathologic correlation. *Radiographics* 15:421-437, 1995.

Cross-Reference

Thoracic Radiology: THE REQUISITES, 2nd ed, pp 188-190.

Comment

Sarcoidosis is a systemic disorder of unknown etiology that is characterized pathologically by widespread non-caseating granulomas. Because this pathologic finding may also be seen in a variety of other conditions, a diagnosis of sarcoidosis requires consistent radiologic, clinical, laboratory, and pathologic findings, as well as exclusion of other entities (especially granulomatous infections).

The chest radiograph is abnormal in approximately 90% of patients with sarcoidosis. Bilateral, symmetric hilar lymph node enlargement is the most common radiographic abnormality and is frequently accompanied by mediastinal lymph node enlargement. Lung parenchymal disease is usually nodular or reticulonodular in appearance, with a predilection for the upper and mid-lung zones.

On CT examination (particularly HRCT), sarcoid granulomas typically appear as small (1- to 2-mm-diameter) nodules, with a characteristic perilymphatic distribution. This distribution includes the peribronchovascular lymphatics, the interlobular septa, and the subpleural lymphatics (peripherally and along the fissures). Approximately 20% of patients with radiographic evidence of interstitial lung disease develop interstitial fibrosis.

Notes

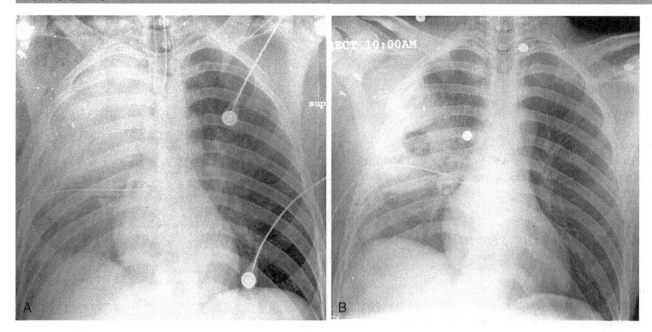

1. What is the most likely cause of parenchymal opacification in this patient who recently sustained a gunshot injury to the right hemithorax?

2. Is contusion an early or late sign of thoracic trauma?

3. When would you expect a contusion to resolve?

4. What other parenchymal injury is evident on the second radiograph of this patient?

Pulmonary Contusion and Laceration

1. Pulmonary contusion.

2. Early (within 6 hours).

3. Within 7 days.

4. Pulmonary laceration.

Reference

Kaewlai R, Avery LL, Asrani AV, Novellline RA: Multidetector CT of blunt thoracic trauma. *Radiographics* 28:1555-1570, 2008.

Cross-Reference

Thoracic Radiology: THE REQUISITES, 2nd ed, pp 168-169.

Comment

Thoracic trauma may result in two forms of lung parenchymal injury: pulmonary contusion and pulmonary laceration. Pulmonary contusion is the most common form of lung injury and represents hemorrhage into the alveoli. On radiographs, pulmonary contusion appears as areas of airspace opacification that are usually in close proximity to the site of blunt trauma, but may also less commonly be observed in the opposite portion of the lung (contrecoup lesion). Thus, the identification of consolidation adjacent to sites of rib fractures or bullet fragments should suggest the diagnosis. The consolidation from contusion typically appears on radiographs within 6 hours of the time of injury, and it usually improves within 24 to 72 hours. The consolidation usually completely resolves within 1 week of onset.

CT may detect pulmonary contusion immediately after injury, before abnormalities are visible radiographically. On CT, areas of contusion may sometimes demonstrate characteristic subpleural sparing of the peripheral 1 to 2 mm of the lungs.

Pulmonary laceration refers to a tear in the lung parenchyma. Such injuries may initially be masked by surrounding contusion. On radiographs of patients with pulmonary laceration injury, you may observe an ovoid cystic lucency that represents a posttraumatic pneumatocele. Such cysts are typically small (5 mm to 1 cm), but larger cysts can be seen in some cases. If the cyst fills with blood, a spherical hematoma is observed. In some cases, the cyst contains air and blood, with a resultant air-fluid level.

Notes

1. Name the location of the intrathoracic, extraalveolar air collection that is evident on the radiograph and CT image.

2. Is there another intrathoracic, extraalveolar air collection evident on the radiograph?

3. What is the most common mechanism for the development of pneumomediastinum?

4. Would you expect pneumomediastinum to change in configuration on a decubitus radiograph?

Pneumomediastinum

1. Pneumomediastinum.

2. Yes—small apical pneumothoraces.

3. Alveolar rupture.

4. No.

Reference
Bejvan SM, Godwin JD: Pneumomediastinum: old signs and new signs. *AJR Am J Roentgenol* 166:1041-1048, 1996.

Cross-Reference
Thoracic Radiology: THE REQUISITES, 2nd ed, p 165.

Comment
There are a variety of causes of pneumomediastinum. Intrathoracic sources include ruptured alveoli, tracheal perforation, and esophageal rupture. Air may also enter the mediastinum from the neck or retroperitoneum.

Alveolar rupture is the most common mechanism of pneumomediastinum and may occur secondary to elevated intraalveolar pressure or damage to alveolar walls. Causes of elevated intraalveolar pressure include airway obstruction (e.g., asthma, foreign body), mechanical ventilation, blunt thoracic trauma (the cause in this case), coughing, Valsalva maneuver, and vomiting. Disorders associated with alveolar wall damage include pneumonia, adult respiratory distress syndrome, emphysema, and interstitial fibrosis.

On radiographs of patients with pneumomediastinum, you will observe lucent streaks of air that surround the mediastinal structures, elevate the mediastinal pleura, and frequently extend into the soft tissues of the neck. In most cases, pneumomediastinum is readily distinguishable from pneumothorax and pneumopericardium. However, when only a small amount of gas is localized adjacent to the heart border, it may be difficult to distinguish these entities. In such cases, a lateral decubitus view may be helpful: unlike pneumothorax and pneumopericardium, pneumomediastinum will not shift in position.

Notes

1. Name four features that are typical of malignant pleural thickening.

2. Which is more common: pleural metastases or malignant mesothelioma?

3. How frequently are pleural calcifications observed on CT scans of patients with malignant mesothelioma?

4. What is the typical latency period between exposure to asbestos and development of malignant mesothelioma?

Malignant Mesothelioma

1. Greater than 1 cm in thickness, nodularity, circumferential growth pattern within the involved hemithorax, and involvement of the mediastinal pleural.

2. Pleural metastases.

3. Approximately 20%.

4. Between 30 and 40 years.

Reference
Miller BH, Rosado-de-Christenson ML, Mason AC, et al: Malignant pleural mesothelioma: radiologic-pathologic correlation. *Radiographics* 16:613-644, 1996.

Cross-Reference
Thoracic Radiology: THE REQUISITES, 2nd ed, pp 392-395.

Comment
Malignant mesothelioma is the most common primary neoplasm of the pleura, but it is a relatively rare entity. In approximately 80% of cases, it affects individuals who have been exposed to asbestos. Males are affected more commonly than females. Presenting symptoms include chest pain and dyspnea.

The most common radiographic finding is the presence of diffuse pleural thickening that is typically nodular and irregular in configuration. Diffuse pleural thickening may be accompanied by a reduction in the size of the affected hemithorax, with associated ipsilateral shift of the mediastinum. Pleural effusion is often present.

CT and MR are superior to radiography in assessing the extent of disease. In many cases, CT and MR play complementary roles in determining resectability and may be used to assess transdiaphragmatic extension, diffuse chest wall invasion, invasion of vital mediastinal structures, vertebral body invasion, direct extension of tumor to the contralateral pleura, and the presence of distant metastases. The presence of one or more of these findings precludes surgical resection.

Patients with limited disease may be considered candidates for attempted surgical cure by extrapleural pneumonectomy. Regardless of therapy, however, malignant mesothelioma is almost always fatal.

Notes

1. Where is the pleural effusion located in the first figure?

2. What is the most sensitive radiographic projection for detecting a pleural effusion?

3. How much pleural fluid must be present in order to observe blunting of the costophrenic angle on the frontal chest radiograph?

4. Name the two most common causes of an exudative pleural effusion.

Subpulmonic Pleural Effusion

1. Subpulmonic space.

2. Lateral decubitus view.

3. At least 200 ml.

4. Infection and neoplasm.

Reference
Stark P: Imaging of pleural effusions in adult. In: Rose BD, Ed. *UpToDate*. Waltham, MA: UpToDate, 2007.

Cross-Reference
Thoracic Radiology: THE REQUISITES, 2nd ed, pp 166-167, 382.

Comment
On an upright chest radiograph, a pleural effusion is usually manifested by the presence of a *meniscus sign,* which refers to a blunted appearance of the costophrenic angle, with a concave upward slope. In general, it requires approximately 200 ml of fluid to blunt the lateral costophrenic angle but only approximately 75 ml of fluid to blunt the posterior costophrenic angle. A lateral decubitus view can demonstrate as little as 5 ml of fluid.

In some patients, a large amount of free-flowing pleural fluid may collect in the subpulmonic space before spilling into the costophrenic angle. In such cases, you may observe a characteristic appearance on the frontal chest radiograph, including an apparent elevation of the hemidiaphragm, flattening of the diaphragm contour medially, and displacement of the peak of the diaphragm laterally. A suspected subpulmonic effusion can be confirmed by obtaining a lateral decubitus radiograph (second figure).

On the basis of laboratory evaluation, pleural effusions can be classified as exudates or transudates. Causes of exudates include infection, infarction, neoplasm, and inflammatory disorders. Causes of transudates include congestive heart failure, low protein level, myxedema, cirrhosis, nephrotic syndrome, and constrictive pericarditis.

Notes

1. What abnormal extraalveolar intrathoracic air collection is evident on this supine chest radiograph?

2. What are the two most common locations of a pneumothorax on a supine radiograph?

3. On a supine radiograph, is an apicolateral visceral pleural line a highly sensitive sign for the diagnosis of pneumothorax?

4. Name at least three radiographic findings associated with a subpulmonic pneumothorax on a supine radiograph.

Pneumothorax on Supine Radiograph

1. Pneumothorax.

2. Anteromedial and subpulmonic.

3. No.

4. Hyperlucent upper abdominal quadrant, deep sulcus sign, sharp diaphragmatic contour, and *double diaphragm sign* (this sign refers to visualization of the anterior and posterior surfaces of the diaphragm).

Reference

Hill JR, Norner PE, Primack SL: ICU imaging. *Clin Chest Med* 29:59-76, 2008.

Cross-Reference

Thoracic Radiology: THE REQUISITES, 2nd ed, pp 388-389.

Comment

A *pneumothorax* is usually readily identifiable on an upright chest radiograph as an apicolateral white line (the visceral pleural line) with an absence of vessels beyond it. However, in the supine position, the apicolateral portion of the lung is no longer the most nondependent portion. Rather, air collects preferentially in the anteromedial and subpulmonic portions of the chest. Only when a large volume of air is present in the pleural space will you visualize an apicolateral pleural line on a supine radiograph. Thus, although highly specific for pneumothorax, this is not a highly sensitive sign on supine radiographs.

The chest radiograph in this case shows several signs associated with a subpulmonic pneumothorax, including a hyperlucent appearance of the right upper quadrant of the abdomen, a deep costophrenic sulcus, and a sharp right hemidiaphragm contour. Also note the sharp outline of the right cardiac and mediastinal contours, findings associated with anteromedial pneumothorax.

Notes

1. Where are these masses located?

2. Which feature is most helpful for differentiating a pleural mass from an extrapleural (chest wall) mass?

3. What are the two most common causes of an extrapleural mass with associated rib destruction in an adult patient?

4. Name two causes of hypervascular chest wall metastases.

Extrapleural Masses Secondary to Metastatic Thyroid Carcinoma

1. Extrapleural (chest wall).

2. The presence of rib abnormalities such as destruction or remodeling suggests an extrapleural location.

3. Metastatic disease and myeloma.

4. Thyroid carcinoma and renal cell carcinoma.

Reference

Reed JC: Chest wall lesions. In: *Chest Radiology: Plain Film Patterns and Differential Diagnoses*, fifth edition. Philadelphia, Mosby, 2003, pp 6-24.

Cross-Reference

Thoracic Radiology: THE REQUISITES, 2nd ed, pp 40-41.

Comment

The chest radiograph shows multiple masses that form obtuse angles with the adjacent chest wall and have incomplete, tapered borders. Such an appearance is typical of an intrathoracic, extrapulmonary location. The identification of rib destruction (best seen on the CT image) confirms that the masses are extrapleural.

In an adult patient, the most common causes of chest wall masses with associated rib destruction are metastatic disease and multiple myeloma. The contrast-enhanced CT image shows intense enhancement of the mass, a finding that is associated with hypervascular metastases. The most common causes for such findings are metastatic thyroid carcinoma and renal cell carcinoma.

Notes

1. What is the location of the confluent opacity in the right hemithorax?

2. What feature of this opacity on the PA projection suggests an extraparenchymal location?

3. What features of this opacity suggest a pleural location on the lateral projection?

4. What is the term used to describe a masslike opacity due to loculated pleural fluid within a fissure?

Loculated Pleural Fluid in the Major Fissure

1. Pleura (the major fissure).

2. Incomplete borders (note the sharp margins infero-medially and the lack of a distinct margin superolaterally).

3. Elliptical configuration and an oblique orientation corresponding to the course of the major fissure.

4. Vanishing tumor, phantom tumor, or pseudotumor.

Reference

Reed JC: Pleural and subpleural opacities. In: *Chest Radiology: Plain Film Patterns and Differential Diagnoses*, fifth edition. Philadelphia, Mosby, 2003, pp 25-46.

Cross-Reference

Thoracic Radiology: THE REQUISITES, 2nd ed, pp 381, 382.

Comment

The chest radiograph in this case demonstrates the characteristic appearance of a loculated pleural fluid collection within the major fissure. Such loculation occurs most commonly in patients with heart failure. Loculated fluid is seen more often in the right lung than in the left, and the minor fissure is more commonly involved than the major fissure. Because of the transient nature of loculated fluid collections, they have been referred to as "vanishing tumors," "phantom tumors," and "pseudotumors." Such terms should be avoided in radiology reports to avoid possible confusion.

When fluid is loculated within the major fissure, it may appear on the PA projection as either a discrete, masslike opacity with incomplete borders (as demonstrated in the first figure) or as a hazy, veil-like opacity. On the lateral radiograph, such a loculated fluid collection appears as a well-marginated, elliptical opacity coursing along the obliquely oriented axis of the major fissure (as demonstrated in the second figure). The rapid onset and resolution of such fluid collections usually allow one to readily distinguish loculated fluid from a solid pleural mass. When the diagnosis is in doubt, a decubitus view may be helpful, because it will demonstrate the free fluid to shift in distribution. CT can readily differentiate pleural fluid collections from solid masses and may be useful in selected "problem" cases in which there is a lack of shift on decubitus radiographs due to loculation.

Notes

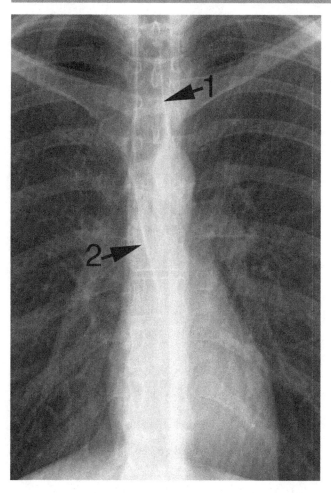

1. Name the mediastinal line that is indicated by the *arrow labeled 2.*

2. How many layers of pleura form this line?

3. Which line extends above the level of the clavicles—the anterior or the posterior junction line?

4. Which line is visualized more frequently—the anterior or the posterior junction line?

Junction Lines

1. Anterior junction line.

2. Four.

3. Posterior junction line *(arrow labeled 1).*

4. Anterior junction line.

Reference

Müller NL, Silva CIS: Normal chest radiograph. In: Silva CIS, Müller NL, Eds. *Imaging of the Chest.* Philadelphia, Saunders, 2008, pp 3-33.

Cross-Reference

Thoracic Radiology: THE REQUISITES, 2nd ed, pp 339, 341.

Comment

The coned-down frontal radiograph demonstrates the normal appearance of the anterior junction line *(arrow labeled 2)* that is formed by the close apposition of the visceral and parietal layers of pleura of both lungs as they approximate anterior to the mediastinum. Similarly, the posterior junction line *(arrow labeled 1)* represents the apposition of pleural layers of both lungs as they approximate posterior to the mediastinum.

The anterior portion of the thorax begins at the thoracic inlet. Thus, the anterior junction line begins at the undersurface of the clavicles. It typically courses obliquely from right to left, as demonstrated in this case. The posterior portion of the thorax extends more superiorly than the anterior portion. Thus, the posterior junction line may be seen above the level of the clavicles, as in this illustration. It typically appears as a straight vertical line, often visible through the tracheal air column.

The identification of a displaced or obliterated junction line can help to identify and localize a mediastinal mass. Displacement of a junction line is also an indicator of volume loss and may accompany atelectasis of a lobe or of an entire lung.

Notes

1. What is the most likely cause of the thickened tracheoesophageal stripe observed on the lateral chest radiograph?

2. What are the major risk factors for developing esophageal carcinoma?

3. What are the two most common cell types of esophageal neoplasm?

4. What is the most common benign esophageal neoplasm?

Esophageal Carcinoma

1. Esophageal carcinoma.

2. Cigarette smoking and alcohol ingestion (additional risk factors include achalasia, preexisting benign stricture, Barrett's esophagus, tylosis, Plummer-Vinson syndrome, and sprue).

3. Squamous cell carcinoma and adenocarcinoma together account for more than 90% of esophageal cancers.

4. Leiomyoma.

Reference

Kim TJ, Kim HY, Lee KW, Kim MS: Multimodality assessment of esophageal cancer: preoperative staging and monitoring of response to therapy. *Radiographics* 29:403-421, 2009.

Cross-Reference

Thoracic Radiology: THE REQUISITES, 2nd ed, pp 364-366.

Comment

The lateral chest radiograph demonstrates abnormal thickening of the tracheoesophageal stripe and anterior displacement of the trachea. A tracheoesophageal stripe that measures more than 5 mm in width should be considered abnormal and usually signifies the presence of esophageal carcinoma. The CT image confirms the presence of esophageal wall thickening. Images below this level (not shown) demonstrated an obstructing esophageal neoplasm.

In patients with esophageal carcinoma, CT can be helpful for assessing the extent of the primary esophageal lesion, identifying nodal spread, and determining extension of the neoplasm beyond the esophagus. CT is often used in conjunction with endoscopic ultrasound and PET for staging purposes.

Although squamous cell carcinoma once represented greater than 90% of all esophageal neoplasms in the United States, there has been a dramatic increase in the incidence of adenocarcinoma. Adenocarcinoma and squamous cell carcinoma now occur with a similar frequency.

Notes

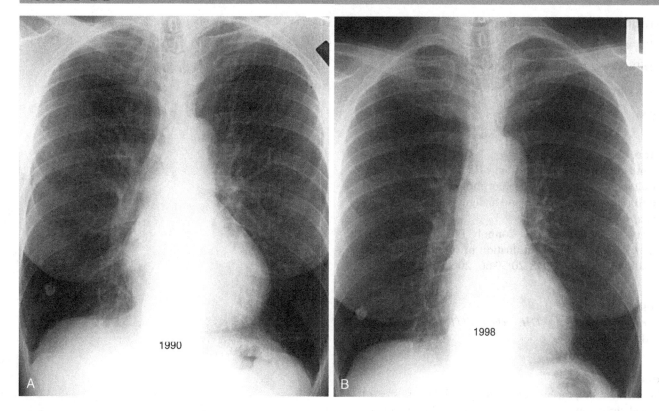

1. Measurements of this nodule show no change in size during the interval between these two radiographs. Is this nodule benign, indeterminate, or malignant?

2. Name at least three benign calcification patterns.

3. Name at least one calcification pattern that is not considered benign.

4. Are follow-up radiographs or CT necessary to further evaluate this nodule?

Benign Calcified Granuloma

1. Benign.

2. Diffuse, central, popcorn, and laminar (concentric).

3. Eccentric; stippled.

4. No.

References

Erasmus JJ, Connoly JE, McAdams HP, Roggli VL: Solitary pulmonary nodules: part I. Morphologic evaluation for differentiation of benign and malignant lesions. *Radiographics* 20:43-58, 2000.

Erasmus JJ, McAdams HP, Connoly JE: Solitary pulmonary nodules: part II. Evaluation of the indeterminate nodule. *Radiographics* 20:59-66, 2000.

Cross-Reference

Thoracic Radiology: THE REQUISITES, 2nd ed, pp 284-286.

Comment

The chest radiographs demonstrate stability in size of a small right lower lobe nodule over an 8-year period. Note the presence of laminar calcification, a recognized benign pattern.

There are two accepted radiographic criteria for a benign solitary pulmonary nodule: (1) lack of interval growth for at least 2 years and (2) identification of a benign calcification pattern within a smoothly margin-ated pulmonary nodule.

Approximately half of all resected solitary pulmonary nodules prove to be benign. Clinical indicators that suggest a benign diagnosis include age younger than 35 years and history of exposure to tuberculosis or residence in an endemic granuloma area. Such indicators are, unfortunately, insufficiently specific to be helpful in most individual cases.

For patients with nodules that do not meet the accepted radiographic criteria for benignancy, noncontrast CT with thin-section imaging is usually the preferred method for further evaluation. CT is more sensitive than conventional radiographs for detecting calcium and fat within a nodule. In certain cases, CT imaging allows a confident diagnosis of a specific benign entity such as granuloma, hamartoma, arteriovenous malformation, pulmonary infarction, mucoid impaction, and pulmonary sequestration.

When CT is nondiagnostic, the method of further evaluation depends on patient characteristics and nodule morphology. Noninvasive imaging modalities include contrast-enhanced CT to assess for abnormal nodule enhancement and 2-[fluorine-18] fluoro-2-deoxy-D-glu-cose (FDG) PET imaging, which relies on abnormal glucose analogue (FDG) uptake to distinguish benign from malignant nodules.

Notes

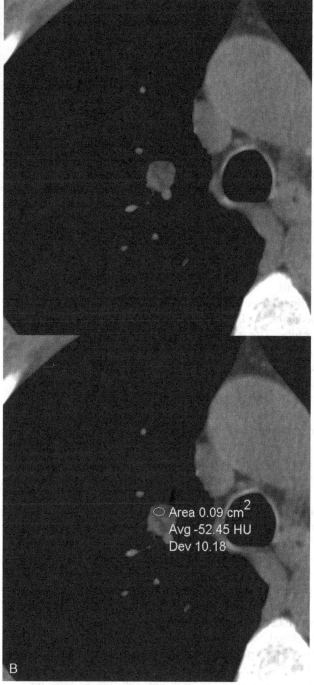

Area 0.09 cm^2
Avg -52.45 HU
Dev 10.18

1. CT density measurements of this nodule revealed areas of low attenuation, measuring approximately −52 Hounsfield units. What type of tissue is associated with this Hounsfield measurement?

2. What is the diagnosis for this solitary pulmonary nodule?

3. Is this a benign or a malignant entity?

4. Are hamartomas always stable in size over time?

Hamartoma

1. Fat.

2. Hamartoma.

3. Benign.

4. No.

Reference

Erasmus JJ, Connolly JE, McAdams HP, Roggli VL: Solitary pulmonary nodules: Part I. Morphologic evaluation for differentiation of benign and malignant lesions. *Radiographics* 20:43-58, 2000.

Cross-Reference

Thoracic Radiology: THE REQUISITES, 2nd ed, pp 253, 254.

Comment

The thin-section CT images demonstrate a well-circumscribed, spherical, solitary pulmonary nodule in the right upper lobe. The nodule contains several low-attenuation areas, which represent focal deposits of fat. The identification of fat deposits (−50 to −150 Hounsfield units) within a pulmonary nodule is diagnostic of a hamartoma, the most common benign pulmonary neoplasm.

A hamartoma is an acquired lesion that represents a disorganized growth of tissue normally found within the lung. Pathologically, the tumors contain cartilage, fibrous tissue, and mature fat cells. Other mesenchymal elements such as bone, vessels, and smooth muscle may also be present.

Affected patients range in age from 30 to 70 years, with a peak incidence observed in the sixth decade of life. There is a slight female predominance. The majority of lesions are detected incidentally on routine chest radiographs of asymptomatic patients. An exception is the presence of an endobronchial hamartoma, which may present with symptoms of airway obstruction.

On imaging studies, hamartomas typically appear as well-defined, solitary, spherical nodules or masses. A characteristic "popcorn" pattern of calcification is identified in approximately 10% to 15% of cases on conventional radiographs and in approximately 25% of cases on CT imaging. Hamartomas typically grow slowly and may rarely be multiple.

Thin-section CT evaluation is more accurate than conventional radiography for diagnosing hamartoma. In the majority of cases, CT will demonstrate one of the following patterns: foci of fat attenuation; a combination of fat and calcification; or lobular ("popcorn") calcification.

Notes

1. Name the pattern of lung opacification observed in the left lower lobe of this patient.

2. What is the term used to describe the air-filled, tubular, branching structures that are visible within the left lower lobe?

3. Name at least three substances that may fill the alveolar spaces and produce airspace opacity.

4. Name the organism that is most frequently associated with lobar pneumonia in the normal (non-immunosuppressed) host.

Left Lower Lobe Pneumonia

1. Alveolar consolidation.

2. Air bronchograms.

3. Water (edema), pus (pneumonia), blood (hemorrhage), cells (bronchioalveolar cell carcinoma), and protein (alveolar proteinosis).

4. *Streptococcus pneumoniae.*

Reference
Gharib AM, Stern EJ: Radiology of pneumonia. *Med Clin North Am* 85:1461-1491, 2001.

Cross-Reference
Thoracic Radiology: THE REQUISITES, 2nd ed, pp 27-28, 80-82.

Comment
The chest radiograph demonstrates the presence of confluent opacification in the left lower lobe with prominent air bronchograms, consistent with alveolar consolidation. This pattern may be caused by the accumulation of edema, pus, hemorrhage, cells, or protein within the alveolar spaces.

Once a pattern of alveolar consolidation has been identified, it is important to determine the distribution and chronicity of the process and correlate the imaging findings with the clinical presentation of the patient.

The distribution of alveolar consolidation is often quite helpful in narrowing the differential diagnosis. For example, the presence of a bilateral, perihilar distribution of alveolar consolidation is most suggestive of hydrostatic pulmonary edema. In contrast, this case demonstrates a striking lobar distribution of consolidation, a pattern that is most commonly associated with pneumonia. The most common organism to produce a lobar pneumonia is *S. pneumoniae*. Other organisms such as *Klebsiella pneumoniae*, *Legionella pneumophila*, and *Mycoplasma pneumoniae* may also produce a lobar consolidation pattern.

With regard to the chronicity of a consolidative pattern, this factor is best determined by comparing the current study with prior chest radiographs. The presence of chronic airspace disease or consolidation is associated with a limited differential diagnosis that includes bronchioloalveolar carcinoma (BAC), alveolar proteinosis, lipoid pneumonia, lymphoma, and the "alveolar" form of sarcoid.

Notes

1. In this patient with a history of Hodgkin's lymphoma, what is the most likely etiology of the paramediastinal lung parenchymal opacification?

2. Is this a common finding in patients who have received mantle radiation therapy for lymphoma?

3. At what time point following completion of radiation therapy is radiation pneumonitis usually detectable by chest radiography?

4. Name the term that is used to describe the presence of dilated bronchi within areas of fibrosis.

Radiation Pneumonitis

1. Radiation pneumonitis.

2. Yes.

3. Approximately 6 to 8 weeks.

4. Traction bronchiectasis.

Reference

Choi YW, Munden RF, Erasmus JJ, et al: Effects of radiation therapy on the lung: radiologic appearances and differential diagnosis. *Radiographics* 24:985-997, 2004.

Cross-Reference

Thoracic Radiology: THE REQUISITES, 2nd ed, pp 277-278, 280.

Comment

The chest radiograph demonstrates a bilateral, paramediastinal distribution of parenchymal opacification with associated air bronchograms. The geographic margins and geometric shape correspond to the field of irradiation.

Radiation pneumonitis and fibrosis are observed in the majority of patients who have received mantle radiation therapy for lymphoma. Radiation pneumonitis is generally observed on chest radiographs within 6 to 8 weeks following completion of treatment, but CT may detect subtle abnormalities earlier than radiography (within a few weeks after completion of treatment). Such opacities are characteristically sharply demarcated and are not limited by anatomic boundaries such as fissures. Fibrosis usually develops within 6 to 12 months following radiation therapy. With time, the parenchymal opacities generally become more linear in configuration and are usually accompanied by volume loss and traction bronchiectasis.

Several methods have been developed to deliver an adequate dose of radiation to tumors while limiting the amount of exposure to normal lung parenchyma. These techniques include limited radiation portals, tangential beams, conformed therapy, and intensity-modulated radiation therapy. These methods may result in variable patterns of radiation-induced lung injury. Knowledge of the temporal relationship and type of therapy can help to distinguish radiation changes from infection and malignancy.

Notes

1. Define the acute respiratory distress syndrome (ARDS).

2. Name at least three common causes.

3. What sign of barotrauma is evident in this patient?

4. What is the distribution of this abnormal, extraalveolar air collection?

Acute Respiratory Distress Syndrome Complicated by Left Anteromedial Pneumothorax From Barotrauma

1. ARDS is a clinical diagnosis of acute respiratory failure characterized by profound hypoxia accompanied by diffuse parenchymal opacification on chest radiography.

2. Sepsis, trauma, severe pneumonia, circulatory shock, aspiration, inhaled toxins, drug overdose, near drowning, and multiple blood transfusions.

3. Pneumothorax.

4. Anteromedial.

Reference
Hansen-Flaschen J, Sietel MD: Acute respiratory distress syndrome: definition; epidemiology; diagnosis; and etiology. In: Rose BD, Ed. *UpToDate*, Waltham, MA, UpToDate, 2008.

Cross-Reference
Thoracic Radiology: THE REQUISITES, 2nd ed, pp 154-155.

Comment
The chest radiograph of a patient who attempted suicide by drug overdose reveals diffuse bilateral lung opacification with prominent air bronchograms. Allowing for portable, supine technique, the heart does not appear enlarged. Note the prominent lucency along the left mediastinal contour, corresponding to an anteromedial left pneumothorax.

ARDS is a severe form of acute lung injury that is thought to encompass a variety of distinct disorders that share common pathophysiologic and clinical features. It may be precipitated by a variety of pulmonary and extrapulmonary conditions, including drug overdose (the cause in this patient).

Because of decreased lung compliance and the need for prolonged mechanical ventilation, patients with ARDS frequently develop barotrauma, including subcutaneous emphysema, pneumothorax, pneumomediastinum, and pulmonary interstitial emphysema.

Notes

1. Name two radiographic signs of bronchiectasis that are present in this case.

2. What is the most likely cause of bronchiectasis that is most severe in the upper lobes?

3. How is this condition inherited?

4. Does this condition ever initially present in adulthood?

Cystic Fibrosis

1. Bronchial wall thickening forming parallel linear opacities ("tram-tracking") and ring shadows.

2. Cystic fibrosis (CF).

3. Autosomal recessive.

4. Yes—occasionally mild forms of CF are first diagnosed in adult patients.

Reference
Webb WR: Radiology of obstructive lung disease. *AJR Am J Roentgenol* 169:637-647, 1997.

Cross-Reference
Thoracic Radiology: THE REQUISITES, 2nd ed, pp 318-319.

Comment
The chest radiograph and coned-down view in this case demonstrate bronchiectasis, manifested by bronchial wall thickening (tram-tracking) and ring shadows (*arrow,* first figure). Although the distribution is diffuse, the lung bases are least involved. The findings are typical of CF, a hereditary disorder characterized by abnormal secretions from exocrine glands, including the airways, pancreas, large bowel, and salivary and sweat glands. The major clinical manifestations of this disorder are chronic pulmonary disease due to bronchiectasis and pancreatic insufficiency.

Although CF is usually diagnosed during infancy or childhood, milder forms of the disease are occasionally first diagnosed in adults. Affected patients are at increased risk for pulmonary infections with a variety of organisms, including *Staphylococcus aureus, Pseudomonas aeruginosa, Haemophilus influenzae,* and *Pseudomonas cepacia.* The last organism is a major cause of infection late in the course of CF. Presenting symptoms of CF are related to recurrent pulmonary infections and include productive cough, wheezing, dyspnea, and hemoptysis. The diagnosis of CF may be confirmed by an abnormal sweat test or molecular biologic testing (polymerase chain reaction).

Classic chest radiographic findings include bronchial wall thickening, saccular spaces due to dilated airways, hyperinflation, and mucoid impaction. Recurrent foci of consolidation and atelectasis are commonly observed. Hilar enlargement is frequently seen in affected adults and may occur secondary to hilar lymph node enlargement or PAH.

Notes

1. Can you reliably distinguish between an infectious and a neoplastic etiology of a cavity based on imaging features alone?

2. Based on the location of this cavity, what is the most important infectious consideration?

3. In addition to infectious and neoplastic causes, what other categories of abnormalities should you consider when a patient presents with one or more cavities?

4. Which cell type of lung cancer is most closely associated with the presence of cavitation?

Cavity Due to Post-primary Tuberculosis

1. No.

2. Post-primary TB.

3. Vasculitis and granulomatoses.

4. Squamous cell carcinoma.

Reference

Reed JC: Solitary localized lucent defect. In: *Chest Radiology: Plain Film Patterns and Differential Diagnoses*, fifth edition. Philadelphia, Mosby–Year Book, 2003, pp 406-426.

Cross-Reference

Thoracic Radiology: THE REQUISITES, 2nd ed, pp 102-104.

Comment

The term *cavity* refers to a lucency located within a nodule, mass, or focus of consolidation. There are a variety of causes, including infection (pyogenic and granulomatous), neoplasm (usually squamous cell), vasculitides and granulomatoses, and rarely, infarction. The most common causes of a solitary cavity are infections and neoplasms.

Certain features can help you determine the likely cause of a cavity, but they are not specific enough to allow you to make a definitive diagnosis in most cases. Features to consider include wall thickness, presence or absence of a fluid level, location, and presence of adjacent lung parenchymal abnormalities. With regard to wall thickness, very thin-walled (<4-mm-diameter) cavities are often benign. In contrast, neoplasms typically demonstrate very thick walls. There is considerable overlap in this feature, however, and it should not be used as a sole criterion. With regard to the presence of a fluid level, it is most often associated with benign nodules; however, fluid levels may occasionally be observed in cavitary neoplasms that have been complicated by secondary infection or hemorrhage. Regarding the location of a cavity, hematogenous cavities often have a lower lobe predominance, reflecting the gravitational distribution of blood flow. Cavities associated with post-primary TB are most commonly located in the apical and posterior segments of the upper lobes and the superior segments of the lower lobes. Primary lung cancer is most common in the upper lobes, but any lobe may be affected. Regarding the presence of adjacent lung abnormalities, the development of a cavity within a preexisting area of consolidation is typical of a lung abscess.

Notes

1. What is the most likely cause for this intracavitary mass?

2. What pleural abnormality frequently accompanies the development of this abnormality?

3. What is the usual treatment for asymptomatic individuals with this finding?

4. Name at least two therapeutic options for patients who develop hemoptysis from this process.

Mycetoma

1. Mycetoma.

2. Pleural thickening.

3. None.

4. Bronchial artery embolization and surgical resection are the most common therapeutic options. Other reported treatments include direct instillation of amphotericin B via a percutaneous catheter into the cavity and systemic antifungal therapy (usually as adjunctive therapy in combination with surgery).

Reference

Franquet T, Müller NL, Giménez A, et al: Spectrum of pulmonary aspergillosis: histologic, clinical, and radiologic findings. *Radiographics* 21:825-837, 2001.

Cross-Reference

Thoracic Radiology: THE REQUISITES, 2nd ed, pp 113-114.

Comment

The chest radiograph and chest CT images demonstrate the presence of an intracavitary left upper lobe mass and apical pleural thickening. The imaging findings are characteristic of an aspergilloma, the most common radiographic form of aspergillosis.

Aspergilloma (also called *mycetoma*) refers to a saprophytic infection that occurs within a preexisting cyst, cavity, bulla, or area of bronchiectasis. Pathologically, the fungus ball is shown to represent a combination of *Aspergillus* hyphae, mucus, and cellular debris.

Patients at risk for aspergilloma formation include those with CF, sarcoidosis, TB, and emphysema. The infection is typically clinically silent for many years. Presenting symptoms may include cough, weight loss, and recurrent hemoptysis. Although hemoptysis is usually minimal, a minority of patients may present with massive, life-threatening hemoptysis. Severe hemoptysis requires therapeutic intervention such as bronchial artery embolization.

Characteristic imaging findings include a round, dependent opacity located within a cavity or thin-walled cyst. The dependent opacity is often heterogeneous due to the presence of multiple linear collections of air, resulting in a "spongelike" appearance. It occurs most commonly in the upper lobes and is frequently accompanied by pleural thickening. In a majority of cases, the fungus ball demonstrates mobility on changes in patient positioning. An aspergilloma is often surrounded by a crescent of air, referred to as the *monad sign*. In a minority of cases, however, the fungus ball may completely fill the cavity, with no visible air between the cavity and the ball.

Notes

1. Name at least four possible causes for a right cardio-phrenic angle mass.

2. Which one of these entities is the diagnosis in this case?

3. Are pericardial cysts more common on the right or the left side?

4. Do pericardial cysts usually communicate with the pericardium?

Pericardial Cyst

1. Pericardial fat pad, pericardial cyst, Morgagni's foramen hernia, lipoma, thymolipoma, and enlarged epicardial lymph nodes.

2. Pericardial cyst.

3. Right side.

4. No.

Reference

Fujimoto K, Müller NL: Anterior mediastinal masses. In: Müller NL, Silva CI, Eds. *Imaging of the Chest*. Philadelphia, Saunders, 2008, p 1517.

Cross-Reference

Thoracic Radiology: THE REQUISITES, 2nd ed, p 361.

Comment

The chest radiograph demonstrates a well-marginated right cardiophrenic angle mass. The majority of causes of a right cardiophrenic angle mass are benign, as listed in Answer 1.

Although the various causes of a right cardiophrenic angle mass may appear similar radiographically, the CT appearances differ depending on the contents of the lesion. The presence of fluid attenuation within a cardiophrenic angle mass is consistent with a pericardial cyst, the diagnosis in this case. Such cysts are attached to the parietal pericardium, but they do not usually communicate with the pericardial space.

The presence of fat attenuation within a cardiophrenic angle mass can be seen in lipoma, thymolipoma, and Morgagni's foramen hernia. Lipomas usually demonstrate homogeneous fat attenuation. Thymolipomas, on the other hand, contain a variable mixture of fat and soft tissue elements. Herniated omental fat can be distinguished by the identification of omental vessels, which appear as serpiginous, tubular soft tissue densities. In many cases, herniated omental fat is also accompanied by bowel and/or liver. Occasionally, herniated bowel is visible radiographically, allowing you to make a specific diagnosis of this entity.

A soft tissue attenuation cardiophrenic angle mass is suggestive of enlarged epicardial lymph nodes. Such nodes are a common site of recurrence in patients with Hodgkin's disease.

Notes

A

B

1. In which segment of the lung is the consolidation located?

2. What numbered bronchopulmonary segments does this correspond to?

3. Name the order of left lower lobe basilar segmental bronchi from lateral to medial on a frontal radiograph.

4. What is the order on the right side?

Pneumonia of the Anteromedial Basal Segment of the Left Lower Lobe

1. Anteromedial segment of the left lower lobe.

2. Segments 7 and 8.

3. Anteromedial, lateral, and posterior (ALP).

4. Anterior, lateral, posterior, and medial.

Reference
Müller NL, Silva CI: Normal chest radiograph. In: Müller NL, Silva CI, Eds. *Imaging of the Chest*. Philadelphia, Saunders, 2008, pp 13-15.

Cross-Reference
Thoracic Radiology: THE REQUISITES, 2nd ed, pp 80-82.

Comment
The frontal radiograph in the first figure demonstrates a subtle focus of parenchymal opacification in the left lower lobe laterally. The focal consolidation is seen in better detail on the lateral radiograph, where it is sharply marginated anteriorly by the major fissure. This location corresponds anatomically to the anteromedial segment of the left lower lobe.

Note the characteristic lateral location of the antero-medial segment on the frontal chest radiograph. The order of the left lower lobe basilar segments on the frontal radiograph (from lateral to medial) is anterome-dial, lateral, and posterior (ALP). In the right lower lobe, the order of the basilar segments (from lateral to medial) is anterior, lateral, posterior, and medial.

Notes

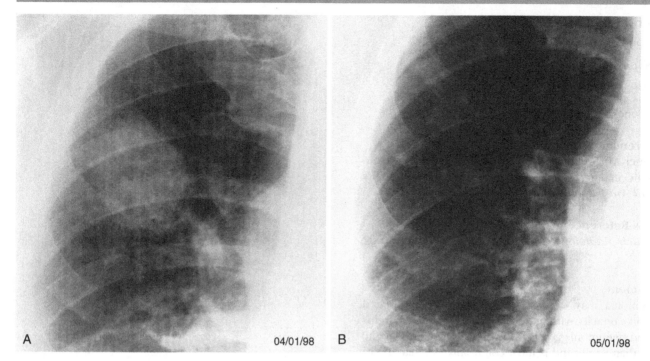

A   04/01/98   B   05/01/98

1. This patient received a course of antibiotics during the 1-month interval between these two radiographs (the first figure preceded the second). What is the likely diagnosis?

2. What organism is most closely associated with a round pneumonia?

3. Are round pneumonias more common in adult or pediatric patients?

4. Based only on the findings in the first figure, what is the most important differential diagnosis to consider?

Round Pneumonia

1. Round pneumonia.

2. *S. pneumoniae*.

3. Pediatric.

4. Bronchogenic carcinoma.

Reference

Wagner AL, Szabunio M, Hazlett KS, Wagner SG: Radiologic manifestations of round pneumonia in adults. *AJR Am J Roentgenol* 170:723-726, 1998.

Cross-Reference

Thoracic Radiology: THE REQUISITES, 2nd ed, pp 82, 83.

Comment

Pneumonia may occasionally manifest as a rounded, masslike opacity with either smooth or irregular margins. Round pneumonia is seen much more frequently in children than adults and is most commonly associated with pneumococcal pneumonia. Round pneumonia has also been associated with a variety of other organisms, including *K. pneumoniae, H. influenzae,* and *Mycobacteriumn tuberculosis,* among others. Round pneumonia has also been described as a manifestation of severe acute respiratory syndrome (SARS) coronavirus infection.

When an adult patient presents with a rounded, masslike opacity, bronchogenic carcinoma is the most important diagnosis to consider. Because neoplasms (especially bronchoalveolar cell carcinoma and lymphoma) may occasionally be associated with air bronchograms, the presence or absence of this finding is not helpful in distinguishing infection from neoplasm. Moreover, only a minority of cases of round pneumonia demonstrate air bronchograms radiographically.

A recent chest radiograph with normal findings and a history of infectious symptoms can aid in the diagnosis of round pneumonia. In adult patients with a suspected diagnosis of round pneumonia, follow-up radiographs following appropriate antibiotic therapy are mandatory. Failure of a rounded opacity to completely resolve following antibiotic therapy generally warrants further evaluation with invasive procedures to exclude neoplasm.

Notes

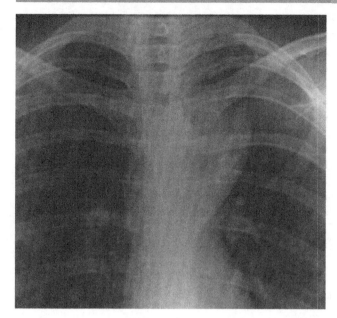

1. Name two features of this mass that are suggestive of a mediastinal location.

2. What osseous abnormality is associated with this mass?

3. Does this osseous finding imply a malignant etiology?

4. What is the most common cause of a posterior mediastinal mass?

Neurogenic Tumor (Ganglioneuroma)

1. Smooth, sharp margins and obtuse angle with the adjacent lung.

2. Rib spreading (left fourth and fifth posterior ribs).

3. No.

4. Neurogenic tumor.

Reference

Duwe BV, Sterman DH, Musani AI: Tumors of the mediastinum. *Chest* 128:2893-2909, 2005.

Cross-Reference

Thoracic Radiology: THE REQUISITES, 2nd ed, pp 362, 363.

Comment

Neurogenic tumors are the most common cause of a posterior mediastinal mass. Such lesions can be classified into three groups: (1) those arising from peripheral nerves (schwannoma, neurofibroma); (2) those arising from the sympathetic chain (ganglioneuroma, ganglioneuroblastoma, neuroblastoma); and (3) those arising from the paraganglia (pheochromocytoma, chemodectoma). The majority of lesions (approximately 70%) are benign.

Neurogenic tumors typically affect patients during the first four decades of life. Most lesions are detected incidentally in asymptomatic patients. Symptomatic lesions typically produce neurologic symptoms such as radicular pain and neuresthesias. Intravertebral extension may result in symptoms of cord compression.

Interestingly, tumors arising from peripheral nerves, such as schwannoma, tend to differ in shape from those arising from the sympathetic chain, such as ganglioneuroma. The former lesions are generally round and the latter are usually fusiform, with a vertical orientation. Note the fusiform shape and vertical orientation of the mass in this case, which is typical of a ganglioneuroma.

Rib abnormalities such as rib spreading and rib erosion are commonly associated with neurogenic tumors and do not imply malignancy. In contrast, the presence of bone destruction is suspicious for malignancy. Vertebral body abnormalities are commonly present. Such abnormalities are best demonstrated on CT examinations. Tumors arising from peripheral nerves are often associated with widening of the neural foramen. In contrast, those lesions arising from the sympathetic chain more often result in anterolateral vertebral body erosion.

On cross-sectional imaging studies, benign neurogenic tumors are usually homogeneous in appearance and have well-defined margins. Malignant lesions are more likely to appear heterogeneous and to demonstrate irregular margins.

Foci of calcification are present in a minority of cases. Such calcifications are more often identified on CT than on chest radiographs. Note the presence of focal calcification on the chest radiograph in this case. Calcification is more commonly observed in tumors arising from the sympathetic chain than in those arising from the peripheral nerves.

Once you have identified a suspected neurogenic tumor on chest radiographs, MRI is generally the preferred cross-sectional imaging modality for further evaluation because of its superb ability to demonstrate intraspinal extension of tumor or the presence of an associated spinal cord abnormality.

Notes

1. Name six causes of total lung atelectasis.

2. In which direction may large pleural effusions shift the mediastinal structures?

3. List three radiographic findings of total lung atelectasis.

4. Name several causes of hemothorax.

Hemothorax

1. Endobronchial tumor, mucus plug, malpositioned endotracheal tube, foreign body, post-traumatic injury, tuberculous stenosis.

2. Toward the contralateral hemithorax.

3. Complete or near-complete opacification of a hemithorax, shift of the mediastinum to the affected side, elevation of the ipsilateral hemidiaphragm (not apparent in acute hemothorax), compensatory overinflation of the contralateral lung, enlargement of retrosternal clear space on lateral radiograph.

4. Trauma (blunt or penetrating), iatrogenic (central venous catheter insertion), complication of surgery, anticoagulation therapy, malignant tumor, catamenial hemothorax.

Reference
Woodring JG, Reed JC: Radiographic manifestations of lobar atelectasis. *J Thorac Imaging* 11:109-144, 1996.

Cross-Reference
Thoracic Radiology: THE REQUISITES, 2nd ed, pp 37, 380.

Comment
Atelectasis of an entire lung may result from mainstem bronchial obstruction of any cause, including central endobronchial tumors, a mucus plug, or the iatrogenic cause of a malpositioned endotracheal tube into the contralateral mainstem bronchus.

Complete atelectasis of either lung typically manifests as complete opacification of the involved hemithorax with mediastinal shift toward the affected lung and compensatory hyperinflation of the contralateral lung. The findings may be misinterpreted as a massive pleural effusion or pneumonia. Central endobronchial tumors that may cause complete lung atelectasis include lung cancer, carcinoid tumors, hamartoma, adenoidcystic carcinoma, mucoepidermoid carcinoma, and metastatic tumors. On frontal chest radiographs, endobronchial tumors may produce the "cut-off" sign with abrupt termination of the air column at the central, proximal margin of the tumor, often manifesting as a sharply defined interface that may be straight or convex in configuration (*left image* in figure).

Large pleural effusion is another cause of complete opacification of a hemithorax and may be distinguished by shift of the mediastinal structures away from the affected hemithorax and toward the contralateral side. In this case, the patient was receiving anticoagulation therapy and presented with right shoulder pain.

Notes

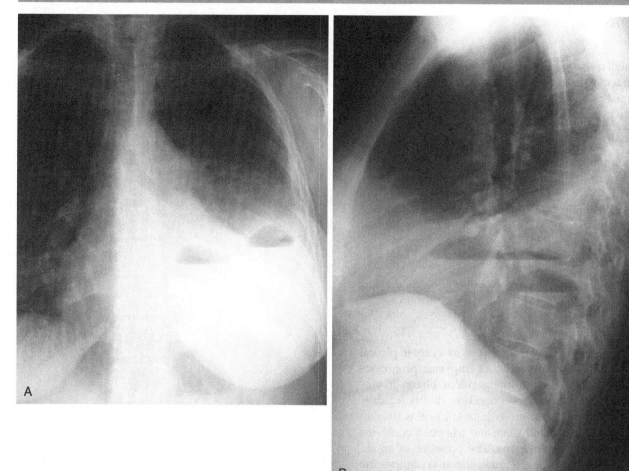

1. Is loculation of a pleural effusion diagnostic of an empyema?

2. List three CT features of empyema.

3. If an air-fluid level within an opacity measures approximately the same on PA and lateral chest radiographs, is the diagnosis more likely to be an empyema or a lung abscess?

4. What is the most likely cause of an air-fluid level within a pleural fluid collection?

Empyema

1. No.

2. Lenticular-shaped fluid collection, obtuse margins at interface with pleural surface, split pleura sign on contrast-enhanced CT, compression of adjacent lung parenchyma.

3. Lung abscess.

4. Bronchopleural fistula.

Reference

Kuhlman JE, Singha NK: Complex disease of the pleural space: radiographic and CT evaluation. *Radiographics* 17:63-79, 1997.

Cross-Reference

Thoracic Radiology: THE REQUISITES, 2nd ed, pp 385-386.

Comment

Initially, empyema typically manifests as a classic pleural effusion on chest radiography. As empyema progresses from an exudative to a fibrinopurulent phase, it may manifest as a loculated fluid collection that is typically lenticular in shape, with more defined margins than an uncomplicated pleural effusion, and will often compress the adjacent lung parenchyma. The presence of an air-fluid level within the pleural fluid collection suggests the presence of a bronchopleural fistula. As in this case, the air-fluid levels may demonstrate a disparity in their lengths when compared on PA and lateral (orthogonal) radiographs, in contradistinction to air-fluid levels associated with a spherical lung abscess, which are typically more equal in length on orthogonal radiography. CT demonstrates these features to better advantage and may show smooth thickening and enhancement of visceral and parietal pleura surrounding the abnormal fluid collection ("split pleura" sign), a finding suggestive of empyema. Additional CT features of empyema include a lenticular-shaped fluid collection, typically forming obtuse margins at its interface with pleural surface, and compression of adjacent lung parenchyma. CT may also demonstrate increased extrapleural fat between the empyema space and the chest wall, particularly if the empyema is chronic. The fat may be increased in attenuation because of surrounding edema. In immune-compromised individuals, or if left untreated, an empyema may drain into the subcutaneous tissues of the chest wall and produce empyema necessitans.

1. Name the two most common causes of rib notching.

2. Which anatomic structures lie along the undersurface of the ribs?

3. What are the osseous manifestations of neurofibromatosis?

4. What is the most common cause of osseous destruction of a rib?

Rib Notching

1. Aortic coarctation, neurofibromatosis.

2. Intercostal artery, vein and nerve.

3. Widened neural foramina, rib erosion (notching), rib spreading, scoliosis, scalloping of posterior aspects of vertebral bodies (dural ectasia).

4. Metastatic disease.

Reference
Boone ML, Swenson BE, Felson B: Rib notching: its many causes. *Am J Roentgenol Radium Ther Nucl Med* 91:1075-1088, 1964.

Cross-Reference
Thoracic Radiology: THE REQUISITES, 2nd ed, pp 362, 363.

Comment
The radiographic finding of *rib notching* refers to focal erosion along the undersurface of one or more ribs. Rib notching was originally thought to be pathognomonic of coarctation of the aorta. However, it is a recognized manifestation of other abnormalities, most of which are related to an artery, vein, or nerve—the major structures found in the intercostal space.

The leading arterial cause of rib notching is coarctation of the aorta with resultant collateral blood flow through dilated intercostal arteries. Other possible arterial causes include entities associated with decreased pulmonary blood supply (i.e., tetralogy of Fallot, pulmonary atresia, Ebstein's malformation, and unilateral absence of the pulmonary artery). The venous system is implicated in rib notching that may occur as a result of superior vena caval obstruction or arteriovenous malformations of the pulmonary or intercostal circulations.

The second most common cause of rib notching is growth of an intercostal neurogenic tumor, particularly neurofibroma, as in this case. Also note the biapical paraspinal masses and nodular soft tissues opacities associated with several lower ribs bilaterally—characteristic findings in neurofibromatosis. The mediastinum may appear widened by paraspinal neurofibromas that extend from the thoracic inlet to the diaphragms. Many ribs may be affected by neurofibromatosis, simulating the rib notching seen in coarctation. Frank destructive changes in a rib should prompt suspicion for malignancy, typically caused by a metastatic lesion.

Fair Game

1. In what mediastinal compartment is this mass located?

2. The majority of anterior mediastinal masses in adult patients arise in which organ?

3. Name at least three causes of thymic masses.

4. How do the metastatic patterns of invasive thymoma and thymic carcinoma differ?

Thymic Mass (Thymic Carcinoma)

1. Anterior.

2. Thymus.

3. Thymoma, thymic hyperplasia, thymolipoma, thymic cyst, thymic carcinoma, and thymic carcinoid.

4. Thymic carcinomas metastasize hematogenously, whereas invasive thymomas typically spread locally within the thoracic cavity (especially along the pleura).

Reference

Nishino M, Ashiku SK, Kocher ON, et al: The thymus: a comprehensive review. *Radiographics* 26:335-348, 2006.

Cross-Reference

Thoracic Radiology: THE REQUISITES, 2nd ed, pp 346-348.

Comment

The differential diagnosis of this poorly marginated, soft tissue attenuation, anterior mediastinal mass includes a thymic neoplasm, lymphoma, and germ cell neoplasm. Lymphoma is typically associated with lymph node enlargement elsewhere, and germ cell neoplasms such as a mature teratoma frequently have evidence of fat attenuation or calcium.

Thymic epithelial neoplasms, most notably thymoma, account for the majority of anterior mediastinal masses in adult patients. Most thymic neoplasms demonstrate well-defined margins on imaging studies. Two notable exceptions are invasive thymoma and thymic carcinoma. *Invasive thymoma* refers to a thymoma that has invaded its fibrous capsule. Such lesions tend to spread locally, with invasion of adjacent mediastinal structures, chest wall invasion, and contiguous spread along the pleural surface (usually unilaterally). Thymic carcinoma is a rare thymic neoplasm that may be indistinguishable from an invasive thymoma on imaging studies unless distant metastases are present. Unlike invasive thymoma, a thymic carcinoma tends to metastasize hematogenously.

Notes

1. What is the differential diagnosis for the subcarinal mass in the first figure?

2. Based on the MRI, what is the most likely diagnosis?

3. Name at least three sites of primary neoplasms that commonly result in metastatic intrathoracic lymphadenopathy.

4. What mediastinal interface is displaced laterally in the first figure?

Subcarinal Lymph Node Enlargement
Secondary to Metastatic Disease

1. Subcarinal lymph node enlargement, bronchogenic cyst, and left atrial enlargement.

2. Subcarinal lymph node enlargement.

3. Genitourinary, head and neck, breast, and skin (melanoma).

4. Azygoesophageal interface.

Reference

Müller NL, Silva CI: Normal computed tomography of the chest. In: Müller NL, Silva CI, Eds. *Imaging of the Chest.* Philadelphia, Saunders, 2008, pp 68-72.

Cross-Reference

Thoracic Radiology: THE REQUISITES, 2nd ed, pp 352-353, 373-375.

Comment

The chest radiograph reveals a subcarinal mass, with associated lateral convex bulging of the azygoesophageal interface. The differential diagnosis of a subcarinal mass includes subcarinal lymph node enlargement, bronchogenic cyst, and left atrial enlargement. The MRI reveals that the mass is not vascular and has intermediate signal intensity similar to that of skeletal muscle. The MR features are thus most suggestive of lymph node enlargement. In this patient, the enlarged nodes were secondary to metastatic disease from a primary renal cell carcinoma.

Enlarged mediastinal lymph nodes may be encountered in a wide variety of neoplastic, infectious, and inflammatory conditions. Neoplastic causes include metastatic disease (from bronchogenic carcinoma or an extrathoracic primary), lymphoma, and leukemia. Infectious causes include tuberculosis (TB), fungal, viral, and bacterial infections. Although lymph node enlargement may be evident on CT images in the latter two entities, it is not usually evident on conventional radiographs. Inflammatory causes include sarcoidosis, Castleman's disease, and angioimmunoblastic lymphadenopathy.

Notes

A

B

1. What term is used to describe the confluent areas of lung opacification observed in these two patients?

2. What pneumoconiosis is associated with this finding?

3. Is this finding typical of the simple or the complicated form of this pneumoconiosis?

4. What term is used to describe the calcification pattern of the lymph nodes in the first figure?

Silicosis

1. Progressive massive fibrosis.

2. Silicosis.

3. Complicated.

4. Eggshell calcification.

Reference

Chong S, Lee KS, Chung MJ, et al: Pneumoconiosis: comparison of imaging and pathologic findings. *Radiographics* 26:59-77, 2006.

Cross-Reference

Thoracic Radiology: THE REQUISITES, 2nd ed, pp 201-205.

Comment

Silicosis is a fibrotic lung disease related to the inhalation of dust containing either free crystalline silica or silicon dioxide. Occupational settings related to silica exposure include heavy metal mining, sandblasting, foundry work, and stone masonry. Silicosis is usually a slowly progressive chronic lung disease with a latency period of at least 20 years.

Chronic silicosis is classified into simple and complicated forms. *Simple silicosis* is asymptomatic and typically presents radiographically with multiple small, nodular opacities, ranging in size from 1 to 10 mm in diameter. The nodules usually have an upper lung zone predominance and frequently calcify. Enlarged nodes are often present and may demonstrate a characteristic peripheral eggshell pattern of calcification, as shown in the first figure.

Complicated silicosis is associated with symptoms and reduced pulmonary function. It is characterized by one or more areas in which silicotic nodules have become confluent, measuring more than 1 cm. Such opacities may be observed in the periphery of the upper lung zone or in the middle lung zone. Over time, these opacities migrate toward the hila, with residual emphysema in the remaining portions of the lungs. In both figures, note the large vertically oriented opacities in the upper and middle lung zones, which are typical of the complicated form of silicosis. As progressive massive fibrosis becomes more extensive, the nodularity in the remaining portions of the lungs usually becomes less apparent.

Notes

1. What is the distribution of lung abnormalities on these high-resolution CT (HRCT) images?

2. Name at least three causes of chronic infiltrative lung disease that are associated with a basilar and subpleural distribution of abnormalities.

3. Which is more common among patients with progressive systemic sclerosis—nonspecific interstitial pneumonia (NSIP) or usual interstitial pneumonia (UIP)?

4. What soft tissue abnormality might you expect to see in a patient with this diagnosis?

Interstitial Lung Disease Secondary to Progressive Systemic Sclerosis (Scleroderma)

1. Subpleural and basilar.

2. Progressive systemic sclerosis (scleroderma).

3. NSIP.

4. Calcinosis.

Reference
Kim EA, Lee KS, Johkoh T, et al: Interstitial lung diseases associated with collagen vascular diseases: radiologic and histopathologic findings. *Radiographics* 22:S151-S165, 2002.

Cross-Reference
Thoracic Radiology: THE REQUISITES, 2nd ed, p 220.

Comment
The HRCT images demonstrate a subpleural distribution of irregular linear opacities, ground-glass attenuation, and traction bronchiolectasis. The last term refers to the small, discrete, cystic lucencies in the lung periphery (best demonstrated in the right lower lobe in the first figure [*arrows*]), which represent dilated bronchioles. A subpleural and basilar predominance of infiltrative lung disease is characteristic of UIP and NSIP.

UIP is characterized histologically by a variegated pattern composed of foci of normal lung, interstitial cellular infiltrates, and intervening zones of active fibrosis and end-stage fibrosis. UIP is associated with a variety of chronic infiltrative lung diseases, including idiopathic pulmonary fibrosis, asbestosis, connective tissue disorders, and drug toxicity. Characteristic HRCT findings in patients with UIP include a subpleural and basilar predominant distribution of irregular linear opacities, ground-glass attenuation, traction bronchiectasis and bronchiolectasis, and honeycombing.

NSIP is characterized by a subpleural and basilar predominant distribution of ground-glass attenuation, irregular linear opacities, and traction bronchiectasis. In contrast to UIP, honeycombing is typically absent in cases of NSIP.

Progressive systemic sclerosis (also referred to as *scleroderma*), is a connective tissue disorder that is characterized by fibrosis and atrophy of numerous organ systems, including the skin, lungs, gastrointestinal tract, heart, and kidneys. Pulmonary manifestations include interstitial fibrosis, pulmonary vascular disease, and pleural thickening. Other common manifestations include esophageal dilation and dysmotility, enlarged mediastinal lymph nodes, and calcinosis in the skin and subcutaneous tissues.

Notes

1. What term is used to describe the combination of a calcified lung nodule and calcified lymph nodes?

2. Are these findings more closely associated with primary or reactivation TB?

3. What does the term *Ghon focus* refer to?

4. Name the two most common radiographic findings associated with primary TB infection.

Ranke Complex

1. Ranke complex.

2. Primary.

3. A lung nodule that occurs at the initial site of parenchymal involvement from primary TB.

4. Parenchymal consolidation and mediastinal and hilar lymph node enlargement.

Reference

Burrill J, Williams CJ, Bain G, et al: Tuberculosis: a radiologic review. *Radiographics* 27:1255-1273, 2007.

Cross-Reference

Thoracic Radiology: THE REQUISITES, 2nd ed, pp 100-102.

Comment

Parenchymal consolidation and mediastinal and hilar lymph node enlargement are the hallmarks of primary TB. The term *Ghon lesion* (or *Ghon focus*) refers to a lung nodule that is a residuum of primary TB. In patients with primary TB and an adequate host immune response, the area of lung consolidation slowly regresses to form a well-circumscribed nodule. Such a nodule may disappear altogether or may remain as a solitary calcified granuloma, referred to as a *Ghon lesion.* Lymph node enlargement, another sign of primary TB infection, also regresses. Residual calcified lymph nodes may be seen, as demonstrated in the aorticopulmonary window and left hilum in this patient.

Notes

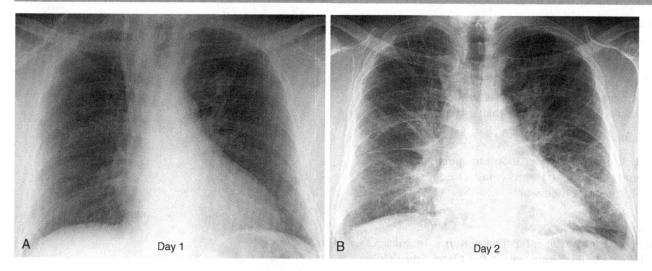

1. What is the most likely cause for the acute interstitial process demonstrated in the second figure?

2. What is the difference between Kerley A lines and Kerley B lines?

3. At approximately what pulmonary venous wedge pressure (PVWP) would you expect to detect Kerley lines?

4. Name at least three radiographic signs of interstitial edema.

Interstitial Edema

1. Interstitial edema.

2. Kerley A lines are centrally located, radiate from the hila, and measure 2 to 6 cm in length; Kerley B lines are peripherally located, usually extend to the pleural surface, and measure less than 2 cm in length.

3. Higher than 17 mm Hg.

4. Peribronchial cuffing, indistinct pulmonary vessels; interlobular septal thickening (Kerley lines), and thickening of the fissures.

Reference

Müller NL, Silva CIS: Interstitial patterns. In: Silva CIS, Müller NL, Eds. *Imaging of the Chest*. Philadelphia, Saunders, 2008, pp 158-199.

Cross-Reference

Thoracic Radiology: THE REQUISITES, 2nd ed, pp 330-332.

Comment

The chest radiograph in the second figure demonstrates several typical findings of interstitial edema, including indistinctness of the pulmonary vessels, peribronchial cuffing, and thickened septal (Kerley) lines. The presence of a recent normal baseline radiograph (first figure) confirms that this is an acute process. Significant ancillary findings include interval slight increase in heart size and increased caliber of upper lobe vessels (cephalization).

Cardiogenic pulmonary edema refers to excess extravascular fluid within the lungs secondary to increased pulmonary microvascular pressure, which is usually due to diseases of the left side of the heart such as left ventricular failure. Cardiogenic pulmonary edema usually follows a typical course. It begins in the interstitial compartment and extends into the alveolar compartment as it increases in severity.

The characteristic radiographic findings of pulmonary venous hypertension and congestive heart failure have been shown to correlate with physiologic parameters such as the PVWP. Normally, the PVWP is lower than 12 mm Hg. As PVWP rises to between 13 and 17 mm Hg, you should expect to see vascular redistribution. At PVWP higher than 17 mm Hg, Kerley lines are usually visible. At PVWP values higher than 20 mm Hg, a right-sided pleural effusion is often evident. When PVWP rises above 25 mm Hg, you should expect to see airspace opacities, usually most prominent in the central, perihilar regions of the lungs.

The chest radiographic features may lag behind the clinical status of the patient as pulmonary edema resolves. Radiographic findings of pulmonary edema may persist despite a return to normal wedge pressure measurements.

Notes

1. What airway abnormality is present in this patient?

2. What is the most common cause of this abnormality?

3. What conventional radiographic sign of bronchiectasis is evident in the lung bases in the first figure?

4. Name at least three CT findings associated with bronchiectasis.

Bronchiectasis in a Patient With Marfan's Syndrome

1. Bronchiectasis.

2. Prior infection.

3. "Tram-tracking" (bronchial wall thickening).

4. Bronchial diameter greater than adjacent arterial diameter, identification of bronchi in the lung periphery, lack of normal bronchial tapering, bronchial wall thickening, and strings or clusters of cysts ± air-fluid levels.

Reference

Javidan-Nejad C, Shall S: Bronchiectasis. *Radiol Clin North Am* 47:289-306, 2009.

Cross-Reference

Thoracic Radiology: THE REQUISITES, 2nd ed, pp 314-321.

Comment

Bronchiectasis is defined as abnormal, irreversible dilation of the bronchi. Bronchiectasis may arise secondary to a wide variety of congenital and acquired abnormalities. Cystic fibrosis is the most common associated congenital abnormality, and prior infection, especially childhood viral illnesses, is the most common acquired abnormality. Bronchiectasis is a rare complication of Marfan's syndrome. Note the characteristic elongated thorax of this patient on the lateral radiograph.

Chest radiographs are frequently normal in patients with mild degrees of bronchiectasis but may occasionally reveal parallel thickened bronchial walls, also referred to as a *tram-track appearance.* With cystic bronchiectasis, radiographs may reveal clusters of air-filled cysts, often with fluid levels. HRCT is highly sensitive and specific for diagnosing bronchiectasis. Findings include a bronchial wall diameter greater than its adjacent artery (resulting in a "signet-ring" sign when the dilated bronchus and accompanying artery are viewed in cross-section), identification of bronchi within the peripheral centimeter of the lung, lack of normal bronchial tapering, bronchial wall thickening, and strings or clusters of cysts. Because bronchial wall thickening may also be seen in other forms or airways disease, it should not be used as a sole criterion for diagnosis bronchiectasis. Complications of bronchiectasis include recurrent infections, hemoptysis, mucoid impaction, and atelectasis (note the left lower lobe atelectasis in the second figure).

Notes

1. What abnormality is depicted on this image?

2. What syndrome is associated with pulmonary arteriovenous malformations (AVMs)?

3. Approximately what percentage of AVMs are
   multiple?

4. Name at least three symptoms or conditions that may
   be associated with a pulmonary AVM.

Arteriovenous Malformation

1. AVM.

2. Hereditary hemorrhagic telangiectasia (HHT), also known as *Osler-Weber-Rendu disease*, which is characterized by telangiectasias, AVMs, and aneurysms in multiple organ systems (including pulmonary, gastrointestinal, cutaneous, and central nervous system).

3. Approximately 30%.

4. Cyanosis, dyspnea, stroke, and brain abscess.

Reference
Lee EY, Boiselle PM, Cleveland RH: Evaluation of congenital lung anomalies. *Radiology* 247:632-648, 2008.

Cross-Reference
Thoracic Radiology: THE REQUISITES, 2nd ed, pp 75-77.

Comment
An AVM represents an abnormal communication between the pulmonary arteries and veins in which there is absence of the capillary network that normally separates these vascular structures. This process results in a right-to-left shunt. Although many patients are asymptomatic at the time of initial presentation, complications of right-to-left shunting include cyanosis, dyspnea, stroke, and brain abscess.

Pulmonary AVMs have a lower lobe predominance, and they often occur in the medial third of the lung. *AVMs* are defined as *simple* when there is a single feeding artery and a single feeding vein; they are *complex* when there are two or more feeding arteries and two or more draining veins.

On chest radiographs, pulmonary AVMs appear as well-defined nodules, which often have lobulated contours. A feeding artery and draining vein can often be identified.

Pulmonary arteriography was historically the modality of choice for defining the number, size, and angioarchitecture of these lesions. However, multidetector CT (MDCT) angiography with multiplanar reformation and three-dimensional reconstructions has been shown to be equivalent to pulmonary arteriography for detection of AVMs and characterization of their angioarchitecture. MDCT is now the imaging study of choice for screening for pulmonary AVMs and may also be used to help select appropriate therapy. Pulmonary AVMs larger than 2 cm are usually treated with endovascular coil embolization or balloon occlusion.

Notes

1. In which mediastinal compartment is this mass located?

2. What is the most likely diagnosis for this mass?

3. How would you characterize this aneurysm according to its shape?

4. Is this a typical location for an aneurysm associated with cystic medial necrosis?

Saccular Aortic Aneurysm

1. Middle.

2. Aortic aneurysm.

3. Saccular.

4. No.

Reference

Agarwal PP, Chughtai A, Matzinger FRK, Kazerooni EA: Multidetector CT of thoracic aortic aneurysms. *Radiographics* 29:537-552, 2009.

Cross-Reference

Thoracic Radiology: THE REQUISITES, 2nd ed, pp 358-359.

Comment

Vascular abnormalities, including aneurysms and vascular variants, are an important cause of middle mediastinal masses. You should consider the diagnosis of an aortic aneurysm whenever you detect a mass in close proximity to the aorta, particularly if a border of the mass is indistinguishable from the aortic contour. The diagnosis can be confirmed with either contrast-enhanced CT or MRI.

A thoracic aortic aneurysm is an abnormal dilation of the aorta. Aortic aneurysms can be classified according to shape, integrity of the aortic wall, and location. With regard to shape, aneurysms may be classified as either saccular or fusiform. *Saccular aneurysms* are characterized by a focal outpouching of the aorta, as demonstrated in the second figure. Such aneurysms are often traumatic or infectious in etiology. *Fusiform aneurysms,* conversely, are characterized by cylindrical dilation of the entire aortic circumference. This configuration is typical of atherosclerotic aneurysms.

Based on the integrity of the aortic wall, aneurysms may be classified as either true or false. *True aneurysms* have an intact aortic wall. The most common cause of a true aneurysm is an atherosclerotic aneurysm. In contrast, *false aneurysms* are associated with a disrupted aortic wall. Examples of false aneurysms include infectious (mycotic) and posttraumatic aneurysms.

Regarding location, aneurysms may be classified as involving primarily the ascending aorta, aortic arch, or descending aorta. Aneurysms that classically involve the ascending aorta include those related to cystic medial necrosis and syphilis. Other causes of aneurysms, including atherosclerotic, mycotic, and posttraumatic etiologies, most often affect the descending thoracic aorta and aortic arch.

Notes

1. What is the differential diagnosis for the wedge-shaped, peripheral consolidation in the left lung in the first figure?

2. What is the significance of the identification of a feeding vessel directed toward the apex of the consolidation?

3. What feature of peripheral consolidations has been described as highly suggestive of pulmonary infarction?

4. What is the estimated prevalence of "incidentally detected" acute pulmonary embolism on contrast-enhanced spiral CT?

Pulmonary Infarction

1. Pulmonary infarct, neoplasm, pneumonia, and hemorrhage.

2. A feeding vessel is a feature that is more typical of pulmonary infarction than the other entities listed in Answer 1.

3. Central lucencies (round foci of hypoattenuation in the central portion of a wedge-shaped opacity).

4. Approximately 1% to 5%.

Reference
Revel MP, Triki R, Chatellier G, et al: Is it possible to recognize pulmonary infarction on multisection CT images? *Radiology* 244:875-882, 2007.

Cross-Reference
Thoracic Radiology: THE REQUISITES, 2nd ed, p 50.

Comment
Pulmonary infarcts typically appear as wedge-shaped foci of consolidation, with their bases abutting the visceral pleura. Like pulmonary emboli, they are usually multiple, and they typically have a basilar predominance.

Revel and colleagues recently assessed the sensitivity and specificity of four findings (triangular shape, vessel sign, central lucencies, and air bronchograms) for distinguishing pulmonary infarction from other causes of peripheral consolidation. Among these features, central lucencies and a feeding vessel (vessel sign) were more commonly associated with pulmonary infarction, with likelihood ratios of 23 and 2.9, respectively. Thus, when you identify a wedge-shaped peripheral area of consolidation with central lucencies and/or a feeding vessel, you should carefully assess for coexisting pulmonary embolism.

Notes

1. What is the differential diagnosis of multiple lung nodules or masses in a patient with acquired immunodeficiency syndrome (AIDS)?

2. In AIDS patients, is the doubling time of nodules a reliable way to differentiate between benign and malignant conditions?

3. What is the most common type of lymphoma to affect patients with AIDS?

4. Is thoracic lymphoma typically nodal or extranodal in AIDS patients?

AIDS-Related Lymphoma

1. Infection (fungal, mycobacterial, septic emboli) and neoplasm (lymphoma and Kaposi's sarcoma).

2. No.

3. Non-Hodgkin's lymphoma.

4. Extranodal.

Reference
Boiselle PM, Aviram G, Fishman JE: Update on lung disease in AIDS. *Semin Roentgenol* 37:54-71, 2002.

Cross-Reference
Thoracic Radiology: THE REQUISITES, 2nd ed, pp 131-133.

Comment
Lymphoma is a common AIDS-related neoplasm, but thoracic involvement is present in only a minority of AIDS patients with non-Hodgkin's lymphoma. Thoracic lymphoma is usually associated with disseminated disease involving the central nervous system, gastrointestinal tract, and bone marrow. In AIDS patients, thoracic lymphoma is typically extranodal. Thus, abnormalities of the lung parenchyma (nodules, masses, interstitial parenchymal opacities) and pleura (effusions) are encountered more frequently than lymph node enlargement.

The differential diagnosis of multiple nodules or masses includes infections and other neoplasms, especially Kaposi's sarcoma. In AIDS-related lymphoma, nodules and masses may grow quite rapidly, with doubling times similar to that of infectious nodules. Thus, a rapid doubling time is not a reliable indicator of benignancy in AIDS patients. With regard to Kaposi's sarcoma, it can be differentiated from lymphoma by its lack of uptake on gallium scans. In contrast, lymphoma is gallium-avid.

Notes

1. Name the three most common sites of traumatic aortic transection.

2. Of those patients who survive to reach the hospital, what is the most common site of injury?

3. Is a mediastinal hematoma specific for aortic injury?

4. Is aortography commonly used to detect aortic injury?

Traumatic Aortic Transection

1. At the level of the ligamentum arteriosum, the aortic root, and the diaphragm.

2. The level of the ligamentum arteriosum.

3. No.

4. No.

Reference
Kaewlai R, Avery LL, Asrani AV, Novelline RA: Multidetector CT of blunt thoracic trauma. *Radiographics* 28:1555-1570, 2008.

Cross-Reference
Thoracic Radiology: THE REQUISITES, 2nd ed, pp 170-175.

Comment
Acute thoracic aortic injury is a serious complication of blunt chest trauma, with an associated high mortality rate. The majority of affected patients die before reaching the hospital, and approximately half of those who present to the hospital die within 1 week without appropriate treatment.

MDCT plays an important role in screening trauma patients for evidence of mediastinal hematoma, an important indirect sign of aortic injury. Although mediastinal hemorrhage is sensitive for detecting aortic injury, it is not very specific. For example, mediastinal hematoma may be associated with injuries to other arterial and venous structures as well as with nonvascular injuries, such as sternal and spinal fractures. When hemorrhage is localized to the periaortic region (first figure), it is more specific for aortic injury. When you identify hemorrhage, you should look carefully for direct signs of aortic injury.

Direct signs of aortic injury include deformity of the aortic contour (second figure), intimal flap (*arrow* in the second figure), intraluminal thrombus, pseudoaneurysm, and frank extravasation of contrast. Multiplanar and three-dimensional reconstructions provide important complementary information to axial CT images including distance of injury from aortic arch branch vessels, length of injury, aortic diameter above and below the site of injury, and coexisting vascular anomalies. Precise characterization of the injury is important for guiding treatment decisions, including surgical repair and stent placement.

Notes

1. What is the most common cause of a thoracic inlet mediastinal mass in an adult patient?

2. What is the most common cause of a thoracic inlet mass in a child?

3. Which CT imaging feature of this mass makes untreated lymphoma a highly unlikely diagnosis?

4. Do thyroid goiters typically enhance with intravenous contrast?

Thyroid Goiter

1. Thyroid goiter.

2. Lymphangioma.

3. The presence of calcification.

4. Yes.

Reference

Reed JC: Anterior mediastinal mass. In: *Chest Radiology: Plain Film Patterns and Differential Diagnoses,* fourth edition. St. Louis, Mosby–Year Book, 1997, pp 107–124.

Cross-Reference

Thoracic Radiology: THE REQUISITES, 2nd ed, pp 351-352.

Comment

A thyroid goiter is the most common cause of a mediastinal mass in the thoracic inlet region in adults. On chest radiographs, a substernal goiter typically presents as a well-defined mass that extends through the thoracic inlet from the neck and is frequently associated with deviation and/or compression of the trachea. On CT imaging, characteristic features include continuity with the cervical thyroid gland, foci of high attenuation on noncontrast images (reflecting the high iodide content of thyroid tissue), focal areas of cysts and calcification, and intense enhancement following intravenous contrast administration.

Although lymphoma may infrequently present as a thoracic inlet mass, calcification is rarely encountered in untreated cases of lymphoma. In contrast, calcification is a common feature of thyroid goiters.

Notes

1. What is the most likely diagnosis?

2. Name four other causes of chronic airspace consolidation.

3. How can you differentiate this entity from the remaining causes of chronic consolidation?

4. What aspirated substance is most closely associated with this entity?

Lipoid Pneumonia

1. Lipoid pneumonia.

2. Bronchioloalveolar carcinoma (BAC), alveolar proteinosis, lymphoma, and "alveolar" sarcoid (not a true alveolar process).

3. Only lipoid pneumonia is characterized by fat density on CT.

4. Mineral oil.

Reference

Rossi SE, Erasmus JJ, Volpacchio M, et al: "Crazy-paving" pattern at thin-section CT of the lungs: radiologic-pathologic overview. *Radiographics* 23:1509-1519, 2003.

Cross-Reference

Thoracic Radiology: THE REQUISITES, 2nd ed, p 237.

Comment

Exogenous lipoid pneumonia is associated with the inadvertent aspiration of oily substances such as mineral oil. On conventional radiographs, lipoid pneumonia typically appears as chronic alveolar consolidation, which is usually most prominent in the lung bases. Lipoid pneumonia infrequently presents as a focal masslike opacity.

On CT examination, the areas of consolidation are characterized by low density, reflecting their fatty composition. The identification of negative CT density numbers in the range of fatty tissue (e.g., –50 to –150 Hounsfield units) within the consolidation is pathognomonic for lipoid pneumonia. Less characteristically, exogenous lipoid pneumonia may manifest on HRCT as geographic ground-glass attenuation with superimposed smooth septal thickening ("crazy paving" pattern) due to intraalveolar and interstitial accumulation of lipid-laden macrophages and hyperplasia of type II pneumocytes along the alveolar lining.

Affected patients are frequently asymptomatic, but a minority of patients present with chronic symptoms of cough and dyspnea. Such symptoms generally resolve once the patient discontinues using the offending substance.

With regard to the differential diagnosis of chronic alveolar consolidation, you may narrow the differential diagnosis by assessing whether the process is focal or diffuse. Focal areas of chronic consolidation may be seen in lipoid pneumonia, BAC) and lymphoma. Diffuse chronic consolidation can be seen in BAC, alveolar proteinosis, alveolar sarcoid, and lipoid pneumonia. Lipoid pneumonia typically has a dependent distribution, which is not typical of other causes of chronic diffuse alveolar consolidation.

Notes

A

B

1. What is the most likely diagnosis?

2. What is the classic triad of abnormalities associated with this entity?

3. Name one other manifestation that affects male patients with this disorder.

4. What is the pattern of inheritance?

Kartagener's Syndrome

1. Kartegener's syndrome.

2. Situs inversus, bronchiectasis, and sinusitis.

3. Infertility.

4. Autosomal recessive.

Reference
Javidan-Nejad C, Bhalla S: Bronchiectasis. *Radiol Clin North Am* 47:289-306, 2009.

Cross-Reference
Thoracic Radiology: THE REQUISITES, 2nd ed, pp 319-320.

Comment
Kartagener's syndrome is a subset of the dyskinetic cilia syndrome, a congenital cause of bronchiectasis that is associated with an autosomal recessive pattern of inheritance. In patients with the dyskinetic cilia syndrome, ciliary function is typically abnormal throughout the body. Thus, affected males are infertile on the basis of immotile sperm.

Patients with Kartagener's syndrome typically present in childhood with symptoms related to bronchitis, sinusitis, and rhinitis. Bronchiectasis usually develops in childhood and young adulthood, and it is associated with recurrent pneumonias. Bronchiectasis is typically less severe than in cases of cystic fibrosis, another congenital cause of bronchiectasis. Interestingly, in patients with Kartagener's syndrome, bronchiectasis has a predilection for the anatomic right middle lobe.

On imaging studies, the combination of situs inversus and bronchiectasis suggests the diagnosis. Ancillary findings may include overinflation of the lungs and focal areas of consolidation and atelectasis.

Notes

1. What is the most likely cause of left upper lobe atelectasis in this patient?

2. Name five tumors that may affect central airways.

3. Based solely on the degree of postobstructive atelectasis present, what is the correct T (tumor) stage for this non–small cell lung cancer (NSCLC)?

4. What is the most likely cell type of lung cancer in this patient?

CASE 52

Left Upper Lobe Collapse Secondary to Lung Cancer

1. Lung cancer.

2. Lung cancer, carcinoid, mucoepidermoid carcinoma, hamartoma, endobronchial metastasis.

3. T2.

4. Squamous cell carcinoma.

References

Kligerman S, Abbott G: Revised TNM staging system for nonsmall cell lung cancer. *AJR Am J Roentgenol* 194:562-573, 2010.

Rami-Porta R, Crowley JJ, Goldstraw P: The revised TNM staging system for lung cancer. *Ann Thorac Cardiovasc Surg* 15:4-9, 2009.

Cross-Reference

Thoracic Radiology: THE REQUISITES, 2nd ed, pp 31-37, 258-261, 263-266.

Comment

The most common cause of complete lobar atelectasis is obstruction of a central bronchus. In an adult patient, lung cancer is the most likely diagnosis.

The tumor-node-metastases (TNM) system for staging lung cancer was revised in 2009. According to this classification system, a centrally obstructing neoplasm with associated postobstructive atelectasis or obstructive pneumonitis that extends to the hilar region but does not involve the entire lung is classified as T2. If the entire lung is involved, then the primary tumor is classified as T3.

Squamous cell carcinomas typically occur in main, segmental, or subsegmental bronchi and grow endobronchially. In contrast, small cell carcinoma is characterized by a submucosal, peribronchial growth pattern and a discrete endobronchial tumor is seldom identified. Small cell carcinoma typically occurs as a large central mass that may narrow the bronchial lumen by extrinsic compression. Adeoncarcinomas of the lung are typically peripheral tumors.

Notes

1. What is the most likely diagnosis?

2. What other organ system is frequently involved by this disorder?

3. Does this patient have the "limited" form of this disorder?

4. What laboratory test is most helpful for confirming this diagnosis?

CASE 53

Wegener's Granulomatosis

1. Wegener's granulomatosis.

2. Renal.

3. No.

4. Cytoplasmic pattern of antineutrophil cytoplasmic autoantibody (cANCA).

Reference

Ananthakrishnan L, Sherma N, Kanne JP: Wegener's granulomatosis in the chest: high-resolution CT findings. *AJR Am J Roentgenol* 192:676-682, 2009.

Cross-Reference

Thoracic Radiology: THE REQUISITES, 2nd ed, p 225.

Comment

Wegener's granulomatosis is a necrotizing vasculitis that classically involves the upper respiratory tract, lungs, and renal glomeruli. A limited form of the disease is largely confined to the lung and is associated with a better prognosis than the classic form.

The thoracic radiologic manifestations of Wegener's granulomatosis are varied, but the most characteristic pattern is that of multiple lung nodules or masses. Such nodules and masses are usually round in configuration, with well-defined margins. They range from 1 or 2 mm to 9 cm in diameter, and cavitation is evident in up to one half of cases. On CT scans, the nodules frequently demonstrate angiocentric features, such as the presence of feeding vessels and a peripheral distribution. The second most common pattern is focal or diffuse alveolar consolidation, which corresponds to the presence of pulmonary hemorrhage.

The diagnosis requires consistent pathologic, radiologic, clinical, and laboratory data. The presence of a cytoplasmic pattern of cANCA, as detected by indirect immunofluorescence of serum, is suggestive of the diagnosis. Treatment with a combination of cyclophosphamide and steroids is successful in most cases.

Notes

1. Which type of infection most commonly presents with multiple poorly defined lung nodules in an immunosuppressed patient?

2. Is the "CT halo sign" (a "halo" of ground-glass opacification surrounding a nodule) specific for *Aspergillus*?

3. What does the ground glass surrounding the nodule represent?

4. Is the CT halo sign typically seen early or late in the course of infection with *Aspergillus*?

Invasive Aspergillus

1. Fungal.

2. No.

3. Hemorrhage.

4. Early.

Reference

Franquet T, Müller NL, Giménez A, et al: Spectrum of pulmonary aspergillosis: histologic, clinical and radiologic findings. *Radiographics* 21:825-837, 2001.

Cross-Reference

Thoracic Radiology: THE REQUISITES, 2nd ed, pp 122-123.

Comment

Invasive pulmonary aspergillosis is the most common fungal infection to affect immunosuppressed patients. It usually affects patients with severe neutropenia, including recent bone marrow transplant recipients, patients with hematologic malignancies, and patients receiving high-dose steroids. Because it is a potentially lethal infection, prompt recognition and treatment are critical.

Aspergillus organisms invade blood vessels, resulting in areas of pulmonary infarction. On chest radiographs, you may observe multiple poorly defined nodular opacities and more confluent areas of consolidation. Foci of consolidation are often wedge-shaped and peripheral in location. When imaged with CT scanning early in the course of infection, the nodules typically demonstrate a halo of ground-glass attenuation, which corresponds to the presence of hemorrhage. In the proper clinical setting (e.g., profound neutropenia), the CT halo sign is highly suggestive of *Aspergillus* infection. However, it is not specific for *Aspergillus*, because it may also be seen in association with other infections (mucormycosis), vasculitides, and hemorrhagic metastases. Later in the course of infection, the nodules may undergo cavitation (the "air crescent sign"). Such cavitation occurs after granulocyte recovery and usually indicates a good prognosis.

Notes

1. Name two infiltrative lung diseases that are associated with a cystic pattern.

2. Describe the typical demographic features (age, sex) of a patient with lymphangioleiomyomatosis (LAM).

3. Is LAM associated with cigarette smoking?

4. Name two pleural complications of LAM.

Lymphangioleiomyomatosis

1. LAM and eosinophilic granuloma.

2. Young (reproductive age) female. Average age at diagnosis is 35 years.

3. No.

4. Pneumothorax and chylothorax.

Reference

McCormack FX: Lymphangioleiomyomatosis: a clinical update. *Chest* 133:507-516, 2008.

Cross-Reference

Thoracic Radiology: THE REQUISITES, 2nd ed, pp 195-196.

Comment

LAM is a rare disease that affects women during their reproductive years. Pathologically, it is characterized by abnormal proliferation of immature smooth muscle cells and the presence of thin-walled lung cysts. Such cysts may rupture, leading to spontaneous pneumothoraces. Lymphatic obstruction may result in chylous pleural effusions.

On conventional radiographs, you may observe a diffuse linear pattern, with preserved or increased lung volumes. Pleural abnormalities, including pneumothorax and pleural effusion, may also be evident. The hallmark of LAM on HRCT is the presence of numerous thin-walled cysts, which are usually regular and uniform in configuration. The intervening lung is typically normal.

The main differential diagnosis is Langerhans cell histiocytosis (LCH). In this disorder, cysts are usually accompanied by small nodules, which may undergo cavitation. Unlike the cysts in LAM, LCH-related cysts have a more variable appearance, with occasional bizarre configurations. Finally, LCH typically spares the costophrenic sulci, whereas LAM has a more diffuse distribution.

Current treatments for LAM include progesterone and, less commonly, oophorectomy. Lung transplantation is a viable option for patients with severe disease. Multicenter trials are under way to assess new molecular-based therapeutic agents.

Notes

1. What is the most likely cause of focal consolidation in a human immunodeficiency virus (HIV)-positive patient?

2. What is the second most common cause?

3. How often does *Pneumocystis jiroveci* pneumonia (PCP) present with this pattern?

4. Are recurrent bacterial pneumonias an AIDS-defining illness?

CASE 56

Community-Acquired Bacterial Pneumonia

1. Community-acquired bacterial pneumonia.

2. TB.

3. In approximately 10% of cases.

4. Yes.

Reference

Boiselle PM, Tocino I, Hooley RJ, et al: Chest radiograph interpretation of *Pneumocystis carinii* pneumonia, bacterial pneumonia, and pulmonary tuberculosis in HIV-positive patients: accuracy, distinguishing features, and mimics. *J Thorac Imaging* 12:47-53, 1997.

Cross-Reference

Thoracic Radiology: THE REQUISITES, 2nd ed, pp 128-131.

Comment

The chest radiograph plays an important role in the evaluation of pulmonary infections in HIV-positive patients. Despite some overlapping features among various infections, chest radiograph pattern recognition can help to narrow the differential diagnosis of pulmonary infections in HIV-positive patients.

With regard to a pattern of focal or lobar consolidation, bacterial pneumonia is the most likely etiology. Bacterial pneumonias are especially common early in the course of HIV infection (CD4 greater than 200/mm^3), and recurrent bacterial pneumonias are now included as an AIDS-defining illness. Commonly encountered bacterial pathogens include *Streptococcus, Haemophilus influenzae, Staphylococcus,* and gram-negative organisms.

When focal or lobar consolidation is accompanied by mediastinal and hilar lymph node enlargement, TB should be considered. Other causes of focal or lobar consolidation are less common, including PCP (which more typically presents as diffuse, bilateral parenchymal opacities) and *Mycobacterium avium-intracellulare* infection.

Notes

1. What infection is most closely associated with low-density nodes with peripheral enhancement?

2. Is lymph node enlargement more common in primary TB or post-primary TB?

3. In patients with primary TB, is lymph node enlargement more common in pediatric or adult patients?

4. Concerning HIV-positive patients and TB, are enlarged mediastinal lymph nodes encountered more commonly in patients with CD4 counts above 200/mm^3 or in patients with CD4 counts below 200/mm^3?

Tuberculosis

1. TB.

2. Primary TB.

3. Pediatric.

4. CD4 counts below $200/mm^3$.

Reference
Burrill J, Williams CJ, Bain G, et al: Tuberculosis: a radiologic review. *Radiographics* 27:1255-1273, 2007.

Cross-Reference
Thoracic Radiology: THE REQUISITES, 2nd ed, pp 100-102, 353.

Comment
Lymph node enlargement is a characteristic feature of primary TB, particularly in children. Lymph node enlargement may occur alone or in association with parenchymal consolidation. On contrast-enhanced CT scans of patients with mediastinal tuberculous lymphadenitis, enlarged nodes often demonstrate a low-density center and peripheral rim enhancement. Histologically, such nodes have been shown to demonstrate central necrosis and a highly vascular, inflammatory capsular reaction.

Although low-density nodes are characteristic of TB, they are not specific for this entity. Such nodes may also be encountered in atypical mycobacterial and fungal infections. Neoplastic lymph nodes (e.g., metastatic seminoma) may also demonstrate this appearance.

With regard to TB in HIV-positive patients, the radiographic appearance varies depending on the patient's CD4 count. In patients with CD4 counts above $200/mm^3$, a post-primary pattern is typically seen. In patients with CD4 counts below $200/mm^3$, you will usually observe a primary pattern, including low-density lymph nodes and consolidation.

Notes

1. In an HIV-positive patient, what is the most likely diagnosis for these findings?

2. Is this infection increasing or decreasing in prevalence among HIV-positive patients in the United States?

3. Below what CD4 count level are patients at risk for *Pneumocystis* pneumonia?

4. Does a normal chest radiograph exclude this infection?

Pneumocystis jiroveci Pneumonia

1. *Pneumocystis jiroveci* pneumonia.

2. Decreasing (secondary to improved prophylaxis and widespread use of highly active antiviral therapy)

3. CD4 less than 200/mm³.

4. No.

Reference

Aviram G, Fishman JE, Boiselle PM: Thoracic infections in human immunodeficiency virus/acquired immune deficiency syndrome. *Semin Roentgenol* 42:23-36, 2007.

Cross-Reference

Thoracic Radiology: THE REQUISITES, 2nd ed, p 128.

Comment

The classic chest radiographic presentation of *Pneumocystis* pneumonia is a bilateral perihilar or diffuse symmetric interstitial pattern, which may be finely granular, reticular, or ground glass in appearance. Importantly, the chest radiograph may be normal at the time of presentation in a significant minority of cases of *Pneumocystis* pneumonia. CT, particularly HRCT, is more sensitive than chest radiographs for detecting *Pneumocystis* pneumonia and thus may be helpful in evaluating symptomatic patients with normal or equivocal radiographic findings.

The classic CT finding in *Pneumocystis* pneumonia is extensive ground-glass attenuation, which corresponds to the presence of intraalveolar exudate, consisting of fluid, organisms, and debris. It is often distributed in a patchy or geographic fashion, with a predilection for the central, perihilar regions of the lungs. Ground-glass attenuation is occasionally accompanied by thickened septal lines, and foci of consolidation may also be evident in severe cases. In up to a third of cases of *Pneumocystis* pneumonia, ground-glass opacities are accompanied by cystic lung disease. Such cysts have an upper lobe predominance and demonstrate varying sizes and wall thicknesses.

Notes

1. Name four benign causes of calcified lymph nodes.

2. In patients with lymphoma, are calcified lymph nodes usually seen before or after radiation therapy?

3. Name a neoplasm that can result in ossified lymph nodes.

4. Which lymph node group is involved in the second figure?

CASE 59

Ossified Lymph Nodes Secondary to Metastatic Osteosarcoma

1. TB, histoplasmosis, sarcoidosis, and silicosis.

2. After.

3. Osteosarcoma.

4. Superior diaphragmatic nodes.

Reference

Johnson GL, Askin FB, Fishman EK: Thoracic involvement from osteosarcoma: typical and atypical CT manifestations. *AJR Am J Roentgenol* 168:347-349, 1997.

Cross-Reference

Thoracic Radiology: THE REQUISITES, 2nd ed, p 353.

Comment

Calcified lymph nodes are usually benign, and they are often related to granulomatous processes, such as TB, histoplasmosis, or sarcoidosis. Neoplastic causes of calcified lymph nodes are less common. They include metastases from mucinous adenocarcinomas and lymphoma. With regard to lymphoma, calcification is frequently seen following radiation therapy, but it is rarely encountered in untreated cases.

Ossified lymph nodes are a rare manifestation of metastatic osteosarcoma. Such nodes appear similar to calcified lymph nodes. In patients with osteosarcoma, the presence of lymph node metastases portends a poor prognosis. Lymphatic involvement is usually accompanied by metastases within the lung, a common site of metastases. Lung metastases frequently demonstrate ossification.

Notes

1. Name two types of infections that may result in rapidly growing nodules in a non-AIDS immunosuppressed patient.

2. What organism is most closely associated with septic infarcts?

3. Name two common sources of septic infarcts.

4. List four CT features of septic infarcts.

Septic Infarcts

1. Fungal (*Aspergillus*, *Mucor*); septic infarcts.

2. *Staphylococcus aureus*.

3. Tricuspid endocarditis (often seen in intravenous drug abusers) and indwelling catheters and prosthetic devices.

4. Poorly defined nodules that frequently cavitate, wedge-shaped foci of consolidation, peripheral and basilar predominance, and feeding vessel.

Reference

Engelke C, Schaefer-Prokop C, Schirg E, et al: High-resolution CT and CT angiography of peripheral pulmonary vascular disorders. *Radiographics* 22:739-764, 2002.

Cross-Reference

Thoracic Radiology: THE REQUISITES, 2nd ed, pp 84, 85.

Comment

Septic infarcts most often originate from right-sided tricuspid endocarditis or from infected thrombi within systemic veins. Other sources include septal defects, central venous catheters, and pacemaker wires. On chest radiographs and CT scans of patients with septic infarcts, you may observe poorly defined nodular opacities and areas of wedge-shaped parenchymal opacification. Such opacities are usually peripheral in location, and they have a predilection for the lower lobes. Cavitation is frequently observed, particularly on CT scans. A characteristic finding on CT scans is the identification of feeding vessels leading to the nodules (*arrows* in the second figure) and wedge-shaped parenchymal opacities. Thus, the CT finding of cavitating nodules with feeding vessels is highly suggestive of septic infarcts.

Notes

1. What postoperative complication is evident in this case (the first radiograph was obtained prior to the second)?

2. Is bronchopleural fistula more common following left- or right-sided pneumonectomy?

3. List four radiographic signs of bronchopleural fistula following pneumonectomy.

4. What nuclear medicine study can be helpful in confirming this diagnosis?

CASE 61

Bronchopleural Fistula

1. Bronchopleural fistula.

2. Right-sided.

3. Failure of the pneumonectomy space to fill with fluid; abrupt decrease in the air-fluid level in the pneumonectomy space; contralateral shift of the mediastinum following pneumonectomy; and identification of air in a previously completely opacified pneumonectomy space.

4. Xenon ventilation study.

Reference

Chae EJ, Seo JB, Kim SY, et al: Radiographic and CT findings of thoracic complications after pneumonectomy. *Radiographics* 26:1449-1468, 2006.

Cross-Reference

Thoracic Radiology: THE REQUISITES, 2nd ed, pp 166-167.

Comment

Bronchopleural fistula is a relatively uncommon but serious complication following pneumonectomy, with a prevalence of up to 5% and a mortality rate of approximately 20%. Major predisposing factors relate to operative causes of bronchial ischemia, such as a long bronchial stump, too proximal a ligation of the bronchial arteries, and disruption of bronchial blood supply from extensive lymph node dissection. Additional risk factors include preoperative radiation therapy, steroid therapy, malnutrition, and resection through tumor or infection.

Following pneumonectomy, the mediastinum is normally shifted toward the side of resection, and the pneumonectomy space gradually fills with fluid over time. Bronchopleural fistula should be considered when any of the following are observed: (1) the pneumonectomy space fails to fill with fluid; (2) there is an abrupt decrease in the air-fluid level in the pneumonectomy space; (3) there is a new collection of air in a previously opacified pneumonectomy space; or (4) there is contralateral shift of the mediastinum. The diagnosis can be confirmed with a xenon ventilation study, which will demonstrate xenon activity in the pneumonectomy space.

Notes

1. What is the most common cell type of bronchogenic carcinoma to present in this location?

2. Does the presence of chest wall invasion make this an inoperable lesion?

3. Name at least two absolute contraindications to surgical resection of superior sulcus tumors.

4. What imaging modality is best suited for determining the resectability of a superior sulcus tumor?

CASE 62

Superior Sulcus Tumor

1. Squamous cell carcinoma.

2. No.

3. Invasion of more than 50% of a vertebral body, brachial plexus invasion above T1 nerve level, esophageal invasion, tracheal invasion.

4. MRI.

References

Bruzzi JF, Komaki R, Walsh GL, et al: Imaging of non-small cell lung cancer of the superior sulcus. Part 1: anatomy, clinical manifestations and management. *Radiographics* 28:551-560, 2008.

Bruzzi JF, Komaki R, Walsh GL, et al: Imaging of non-small cell lung cancer of the superior sulcus. Part 2: initial staging and assessment of respectability and therapeutic response. *Radiographics* 28:561-572, 2008.

Cross-Reference
Thoracic Radiology: THE REQUISITES, 2nd ed, p 265.

Comment

A lung cancer arising at the extreme apex of the lung is referred to as a *superior sulcus tumor*. Affected patients typically present with symptoms of shoulder pain, Horner's syndrome (ptosis, miosis, anhidrosis), and weakness and atrophy of intrinsic muscles of the hand.

MRI is more accurate than CT for determining the resectability of a superior sulcus tumor owing to its superior ability to evaluate tumor extension in the neural foramina, spinal cord, and brachial plexus. PET-CT allows for detection of nodal and distant metastases and is thus helpful for staging.

In this case, note the presence of rib destruction adjacent to the mass (best visualized on the coned-down image), indicative of chest wall invasion. Chest wall invasion is an important preoperative finding, but it does not preclude surgical resection of a superior sulcus tumor.

Operable candidates are usually treated with preoperative radiation and chemotherapy followed by surgery with chest wall resection.

Notes

A   B

1. What is the most likely cause for these HRCT findings?

2. Approximately what percentage of patients with this disorder are cigarette smokers?

3. In patients with this disorder, which portion of the lungs is usually spared?

4. Would you expect this patient to have diminished lung volumes?

Pulmonary Langerhans Cell Histiocytosis (LCH)

1. Pulmonary LCH.

2. Approximately 90%.

3. Lung bases and costophrenic angles.

4. No.

Reference

Abbott GF, Rosado-de-Christenson ML, Franks TJ, et al: From the archives of the AFIP: pulmonary Langerhans cell histiocytosis. *Radiographics* 24:821-841, 2004.

Cross-Reference

Thoracic Radiology: THE REQUISITES, 2nd ed, pp 196-198.

Comment

Pulmonary Langerhans cell histiocytosis (PLCH) is an uncommon idiopathic disorder characterized histologically by the benign proliferation of mature histiocytes. In its early stages, PLCH is characterized by the presence of multiple granulomatous nodules, which are often peribronchiolar in distribution. In later stages of the disease, the nodules are replaced by cysts.

Affected patients are usually young and middle-aged adults, and there is a strong association with cigarette smoking. Symptoms include dyspnea and dry cough.

On conventional radiographs, PLCH manifests as a reticulonodular pattern, with the upper lobes affected to a greater degree than the lower lobes. The lung bases and costophrenic angles are typically spared. Lung volumes are usually normal or increased.

HRCT demonstrates small irregular nodules that are typically centrilobular and peribronchiolar in distribution. Such nodules may undergo cavitation, and may eventually form thin-walled cysts. Cysts associated with PLCH are less uniform in appearance than cysts associated with LAM. Because nodules are not a feature of LAM, the identification of both nodules and cysts should suggest the diagnosis of PLCH.

Notes

A

B

1. Name three possible diagnoses for the chest radiograph findings in this patient with breast cancer who is receiving chemotherapy.

2. Based on the HRCT findings, which diagnosis is most likely?

3. Name four sites of primary malignant neoplasms that are commonly associated with lymphangitic carcinomatosis.

4. Which primary neoplasm is most closely associated with a unilateral distribution of lymphangitic carcinomatosis?

Lymphangitic Carcinomatosis

1. Lymphangitic carcinomatosis, atypical infection, and drug toxicity.

2. Lymphangitic carcinomatosis.

3. Colon, lung, breast, and stomach.

4. Lung.

Reference

Müller NL, Silva CIS: Pulmonary metastases. In: Silva CIS, Müller NL, Eds. *Imaging of the Chest.* Philadelphia, Saunders, 2008, pp 568-581.

Cross-Reference

Thoracic Radiology: THE REQUISITES, 2nd ed, pp 190-192.

Comment

Pulmonary lymphangitic carcinomatosis refers to tumor growth within the lymphatics of the lungs. Interestingly, most lymphangitic metastases are thought to arise from hematogenous spread. Lymphangitic carcinomatosis occurs most commonly in patients with carcinoma of the colon, lung, breast, and stomach and adenocarcinoma of unknown primary.

The chest radiographic findings of lymphangitic carcinomatosis are nonspecific. They include diffuse reticulonodular or linear opacities, septal lines, hilar and mediastinal lymph node enlargement, and pleural effusions.

The HRCT findings of lymphangitic carcinomatosis are more specific. The observed abnormalities reflect the distribution of lymphatics within the lung: (1) smooth or nodular axial interstitial thickening along the bronchovascular bundles; (2) smooth or nodular interlobular septal thickening; (3) smooth or nodular thickening of the fissures; and (4) identification of polygonal structures (secondary pulmonary lobules). An important ancillary observation is the preservation of normal lung architecture.

Notes

1. What is the most likely diagnosis for these imaging findings?

2. What are "satellite" nodules?

3. What is their significance?

4. What are the most common sites for post-primary TB in the lung?

CASE 65

Reactivation TB

1. TB.

2. Small, often rounded, opacities that lie in close proximity to a larger nodule or mass.

3. They are more suggestive of an infectious process, such as TB, than a lung carcinoma.

4. Apical and posterior segments of the upper lobes and superior segments of the lower lobes.

Reference

Lee JY, Lee KS, Jung KJ, et al: Pulmonary tuberculosis: CT and pathologic correlation. *J Comput Assist Tomogr* 24:691-698, 2000.

Cross-Reference

Thoracic Radiology: THE REQUISITES, 2nd ed, pp 102-104.

Comment

The chest radiograph demonstrates a poorly marginated mass in the right lung apex, without evidence of calcification. CT is often helpful to further characterize a lung nodule or mass. In this case, CT reveals a focus of cavitation that is not apparent on the conventional radiograph. There are also two important ancillary findings on the CT image. First, there are several small nodules adjacent to the mass. Such nodules are referred to as *satellite nodules,* and their presence suggests an infectious etiology, such as TB, rather than a lung carcinoma. However, the term *satellite nodules* may also be used to describe foci of malignancy within the primary tumor lobe. Thus, satellite nodules are not pathognomonic for infection. Second, note the presence of numerous small, centrilobular, linear and branching, Y- and V-shaped opacities, a pattern that is also referred to as *tree-in-bud*. This pattern is often associated with bronchogenic spread of TB, a type of dissemination that occurs when a cavity erodes into an adjacent airway. Thus, the combination of an apical lung cavity, satellite nodules, and a tree-in-bud pattern is highly suggestive of post-primary TB.

Notes

1. What is the most likely cause of the precarinal and right hilar masses?

2. Do MRI signal characteristics of lymph nodes effectively distinguish between benign and malignant lymph nodes?

3. Is MRI more accurate than CT in the assessment of mediastinal lymph nodes in patients with lung cancer?

4. Which imaging test is more accurate than MRI and CT in the assessment at mediastinal lymph nodes in patients with lung cancer?

Mediastinal and Hilar Lymph Node Enlargement in a Patient With Primary Lung Cancer

1. Mediastinal and hilar lymph node enlargement.

2. No.

3. No.

4. FDG–PET imaging.

Reference

Lardinois D, Weder W, Hany TF, et al: Staging of non-small-cell lung cancer with integrated positron-emission tomography and computed tomography. *N Engl J Med* 348:2500-2507, 2003.

Cross-Reference

Thoracic Radiology: THE REQUISITES, 2nd ed, pp 266-268, 352-353.

Comment

Lymph node enlargement is a common cause of a mediastinal or hilar mass and should be suspected whenever a spherical or ovoid mass or masses are identified within a known anatomic lymph node location. There are a variety of infectious, inflammatory, and neoplastic causes of thoracic lymph node enlargement.

Neoplastic etiologies include primary lung cancer, metastatic disease, and lymphoma. This patient has a primary lung cancer in the right upper lobe (not shown on these images), and the lymph nodes were proved malignant at biopsy.

Both CT and MRI rely on anatomic features of lymph nodes, most notably lymph node size (short axis larger than 1 cm), to distinguish between malignant and benign lymph nodes. This strategy is limited by a low sensitivity and specificity. Thus, in patients with primary lung cancer, enlarged nodes must be biopsied for staging purposes. FDG-PET imaging, which relies upon metabolic (glucose metabolism) rather than anatomic features, is the most accurate noninvasive imaging test for assessing mediastinal lymph nodes. The accuracy of FDG-PET can be further enhanced by using an integrated PET-CT scanner, which improves visual quality and quantitative accuracy of PET images, while optimizing anatomic-metabolic correlation.

Notes

A

B

1. What is the cause of diffuse mediastinal widening in this patient?

2. Does this disorder require therapy?

3. Name three risk factors for developing this condition.

4. Where does excess fat usually accumulate in patients with this condition?

Mediastinal Lipomatosis

1. Mediastinal lipomatosis.

2. No.

3. Cushing's syndrome, steroid therapy, and obesity.

4. Anterior and superior mediastinum, cardiophrenic angles, and paravertebral and retrocrural regions.

Reference
Boiselle PM, Rosado-de-Christenson ML: Fat attenuation lesions of the mediastinum. *J Comput Assist Tomogr* 25:881-889, 2001.

Cross-Reference
Thoracic Radiology: THE REQUISITES, 2nd ed, pp 369-370.

Comment
The chest radiograph demonstrates a right upper lobe pneumonia and diffuse mediastinal widening. There are a variety of causes of mediastinal widening, including mediastinal lipomatosis, mediastinitis, diffuse mediastinal lymphadenopathy, and mediastinal hemorrhage. The widened mediastinum is relatively symmetric in appearance, and there is no deviation of the trachea. Such features are typical of mediastinal lipomatosis, but a definitive diagnosis requires demonstration of fat by CT or MRI. The CT image confirms the diagnosis of mediastinal lipomatosis.

Mediastinal lipomatosis refers to the diffuse accumulation of excess unencapsulated fat within the mediastinum. Fat accumulation is usually most prominent in the anterior and superior portions of the mediastinum. Fat may also accumulate in other parts of the mediastinum, including the cardiophrenic angles and the paravertebral region. An important diagnostic feature is the homogeneous appearance of the mediastinal fat. A heterogeneous appearance should raise the suspicion of another superimposed process, such as mediastinal hemorrhage or neoplastic infiltration of the mediastinal fat.

Notes

1. What congenital vascular abnormality is evident in this case?

2. Which mediastinal interface is typically displaced in patients with this condition?

3. Name an associated extravascular abnormality that is present on the CT image of the abdomen.

4. Name at least two additional causes of azygos vein enlargement.

Azygos Continuation of the Inferior Vena Cava

1. Azygos continuation of the inferior vena cava.

2. Azygoesophageal interface.

3. Polysplenia.

4. Obstruction of the vena cava, tricuspid insufficiency, and right-sided heart failure.

Reference

Kandpal H, Sharma R, Gamangatti S, et al: Imaging the inferior vena cava: a road less traveled. *Radiographics* 28:669-689, 2008.

Cross-Reference

Thoracic Radiology: THE REQUISITES, 2nd ed, pp 364, 365.

Comment

The chest radiograph and thoracic CT image demonstrate marked distention of the arch of the azygos vein. The abdominal CT image shows dilation of the retrocrural portion of the azygos vein *(arrow)* and absence of a definable inferior vena cava. The constellation of findings is diagnostic of azygos continuation of the inferior vena cava, a congenital anomaly that is associated with both the asplenia and the polysplenia syndromes. Note multiple spleens in the left upper quadrant of the abdomen on the abdominal CT image.

On chest radiographs of affected patients, you will observe widening of the azygos arch contour and displacement of the azygoesophageal recess below this level. CT can confirm the diagnosis by demonstrating absence of a definable inferior vena cava. CT is also helpful in excluding other causes of azygos vein distention such as obstruction of the vena cava.

Knowledge of this congenital anomaly is important preoperatively for planning cardiopulmonary bypass surgery and may also help to avoid difficulties at cardiac catheterization.

Notes

1. How would you describe the margins of this nodule?

2. Precontrast and 1-minute postcontrast images demonstrate nodule enhancement of 35 Hounsfield units. Is this degree of enhancement diagnostic of a benign entity?

3. Which noninvasive test has a higher specificity for malignancy: FDG-PET or CT pulmonary nodule enhancement?

4. Does CT pulmonary nodule enhancement have a high or low negative predictive value for malignancy?

CT Pulmonary Nodule Enhancement

1. Lobulated.

2. No.

3. FDG-PET.

4. High negative predictive value.

Reference

Swensen SJ, Viggiano RW, Midthun DE, et al: Lung nodule enhancement at CT: multicenter study. *Radiology* 214:73-80, 2000.

Cross-Reference

Thoracic Radiology: THE REQUISITES, 2nd ed, pp 284-286.

Comment

The CT images demonstrate a lung nodule with lobulated margins, which enhances by 35 Hounsfield units. The degree of enhancement is greater than the 15 Hounsfield unit threshold for this test and is thus of concern for a malignant process.

CT pulmonary nodule enhancement is a relatively new, noninvasive technique that relies on the principle that malignant nodules are generally more vascular than benign nodules, such as granulomas. This technique requires meticulous attention to the study protocol described by Swensen and colleagues. The protocol employs the use of serial spiral CT acquisitions (3 mm collimation) before and at four sequential 1-minute intervals following the intravenous administration of contrast. Nodule enhancement values are obtained by placing a region of interest measurement within the nodule center. Enhancement less than 15 Hounsfield units is highly predictive of a benign process (negative predictive value for malignancy is 96%). Enhancement greater than 15 Hounsfield units is of concern for malignancy, but the specificity is only moderate (58%). Such enhancing nodules generally require further assessment, such as biopsy or surgical resection.

Because of the need for multiple imaging acquisitions and close monitoring of the scanning and measurement protocols, this technique has not gained widespread use in clinical practice. However, recent technical advances in dual-energy CT, which allow measurement of the degree of nodule enhancement from a single CT acquisition, have the potential to expand the clinical use of CT nodule enhancement in differentiating between benign and malignant lung nodules.

Notes

1. Which hemidiaphragm is more often affected by traumatic rupture, the left or the right?

2. What are the two most common causes of diaphragm rupture?

3. In patients with traumatic rupture of the left hemidiaphragm, which organ is most commonly herniated?

4. Name five radiographic signs of left hemidiaphragm rupture.

Traumatic Rupture of the Left Hemidiaphragm

1. Left.

2. Blunt trauma and penetrating injury.

3. Stomach.

4. Nasogastric tube coiled in the thorax, apparent elevation of the hemidiaphragm with loss of its normal dome shape, changing hemidiaphragm levels on serial radiographs, contralateral mediastinal shift, and left pleural effusion.

Reference

Kaewlai R, Avery LL, Asrani AV, Novelline RA: Multidetector CT of blunt thoracic trauma. *Radiographics* 28:1555-1570, 2008.

Cross-Reference

Thoracic Radiology: THE REQUISITES, 2nd ed, pp 169-170, 173-175.

Comment

Diaphragmatic rupture is an uncommon but serious complication of blunt and penetrating trauma. The left hemidiaphragm is affected more often than the right side. The left-sided predominance is thought to be secondary to two factors: a protective effect from the liver on the right side and relative weakness of the left hemidiaphragm compared with the right.

Because of the morbidity and mortality from associated bowel obstruction and strangulation, a prompt diagnosis of diaphragm rupture is important. Unfortunately, however, the diagnosis is often delayed. You should suspect this diagnosis when you observe apparent elevation of a hemidiaphragm, changing hemidiaphragm levels on serial radiographs, or an unusual contour of the hemidiaphragm. A more specific finding is the identification of stomach or bowel in the thorax. CT or MRI can confirm the diagnosis. Although the direct multiplanar imaging capability of MRI was previously a major advantage compared with CT, the high-quality multiplanar reformations that can now be obtained with thin-section MDCT scanners allow for improved sensitivity and specificity of diagnosing diaphragmatic injury using CT. Because MDCT is better suited to evaluating clinically unstable patients than MRI, CT is currently the preferred imaging test for suspected diaphragm injury in the acute trauma setting.

Notes

1. What skeletal injury is evident on these CT images?

2. Which is more common—anterior or posterior dislocation?

3. Name a potential complication of posterior dislocation.

4. What is the best imaging test for establishing or confirming a diagnosis of sternoclavicular joint dislocation?

Posterior Sternoclavicular Joint Dislocation

1. Left posterior sternoclavicular joint dislocation.

2. Posterior.

3. Injury to the brachiocephalic or subclavian veins. Less commonly, injury to the trachea or esophagus.

4. CT.

Reference

Kaewlai R, Avery LL, Asrani AV, Novelline RA: Multidetector CT of blunt thoracic trauma. *Radiographics* 28:1555-1570, 2008.

Cross-Reference

None.

Comment

Sternoclavicular joint dislocation is a relatively uncommon but potentially serious injury that is usually associated with massive direct trauma to the anterior chest wall. Affected patients typically present with a large hematoma of the upper anterior chest wall and asymmetry of the clavicles on palpation (especially in the setting of an anterior dislocation).

The diagnosis can be difficult to make on portable chest radiographs, because only minimal displacement is usually evident on such studies. Moreover, the sternoclavicular joints are often altered in appearance radiographically on the basis of patient rotation. When this injury is suspected on the basis of clinical or radiographic findings, a limited CT study through the level of the sternoclavicular joints can readily establish the diagnosis. In the setting of a posterior dislocation, contrast-enhanced CT also provides an assessment of the brachiocephalic and subclavian veins for signs of injury.

Notes

1. Is pulmonary embolus the most common cause of unilateral absent perfusion on a ventilation-perfusion (V̇/Q̇) scan?

2. What is the cause in this case?

3. What entities are associated with ascending aortic aneurysms?

4. What other aortic abnormality can result in this scintigraphic appearance?

Right Pulmonary Artery Compression by Ascending Aortic Aneurysm

1. No.

2. Ascending aortic aneurysm.

3. Connective tissue disorders (Marfan's and Ehlers-Danlos syndromes) and syphilis.

4. Aortic dissection.

Reference

Pickhardt PJ, Fischer KC: Unilateral hypoperfusion or absent perfusion on pulmonary scintigraphy: differential diagnosis. *AJR Am J Roentgenol* 171:145-150, 1998.

Cross-Reference

Thoracic Radiology: THE REQUISITES, 2nd ed, pp 358-359.

Comment

A variety of entities may result in the presence of unilateral absence of perfusion on pulmonary scintigraphy scans. Interestingly, thromboembolism accounts for only a minority of such cases. Nonthromboembolic causes include mediastinal and hilar masses, ascending aortic aneurysm and dissection, pulmonary artery hypoplasia and agenesis, pulmonary artery sarcoma, and pneumonectomy. When confronted with this pattern on a pulmonary scintigraphy study, you should carefully assess the chest radiograph for the presence of a nonthromboembolic cause, such as a central mass. CT is often helpful for further evaluation, because it can readily distinguish between an intrinsic filling defect of the pulmonary artery and an extrinsic compression of the vessel.

In this case, absent perfusion to the right lung is caused by severe compression of the right pulmonary artery by an ascending aortic aneurysm. Ascending aortic aneurysms are usually associated with connective tissue disorders such as Marfan's and Ehlers-Danlos syndromes. Syphilis is an infrequent cause of ascending aortic aneurysm. Right pulmonary artery compression is an uncommon complication of ascending aortic aneurysm. More common complications include rupture, dissection, aortic insufficiency, and pericardial tamponade.

Notes

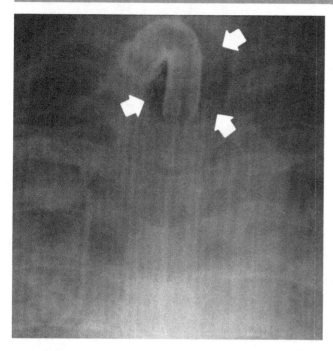

1. What does the circular lucency *(arrows)* adjacent to the tracheostomy tube represent?

2. Name at least two potential complications of an over-inflated tracheostomy tube or endotracheal tube cuff.

3. Name two types of fistulas that may occur as a tracheostomy tube complication.

4. What is the ideal location for the tip of a tracheostomy tube?

Overinflated Tracheostomy Tube Cuff

1. An overinflated tracheostomy tube cuff.

2. Tracheal stricture, tracheomalacia, tracheal rupture, and tracheoesophageal fistula.

3. Tracheoesophageal and tracheoarterial.

4. The tip should ideally be positioned halfway between the stoma and the carina.

Reference

Sun M, Ernst A, Boiselle PM: MDCT of the central airways: comparison with bronchoscopy in the evaluation of complications of endotracheal and tracheostomy tubes. *J Thorac Imaging* 22:136-142, 2007.

Cross-Reference

Thoracic Radiology: THE REQUISITES, 2nd ed, pp 292-294.

Comment

A tracheostomy tube is usually placed for long-term ventilatory support or to establish an airway distal to the presence of a laryngeal obstruction. Most long-term complications of intubation relate to cuff injury. In recent years, the advent of low-pressure, high-volume cuffs has been associated with a decreased rate of cuff complications.

If the cuff is overinflated, blood supply to the mucosa of the trachea is compromised, leading to ischemic necrosis. Late complications of ischemic necrosis include tracheal stricture and tracheomalacia.

A second mechanism of airway injury relates to abnormal angulation of the tube. This problem occurs more frequently with tracheostomy tubes than with endotracheal tubes. Angulation of the tube can result in erosion, ulceration, and eventual perforation of the tracheal wall. Posterior angulation can lead to a tracheoesophageal fistula, and anterolateral angulation can result in a tracheoarterial fistula with either the innominate or the carotid artery. Rarely, an overinflated cuff can directly erode a vessel and result in a tracheoarterial fistula. In this particular case, an overinflated cuff resulted in a tracheocarotid fistula, which proved fatal.

MDCT is highly accurate for detecting complications of endotracheal and tracheostomy tubes, especially when axial CT images are combined with multiplanar and three-dimensional reconstructions.

Notes

1. What is the most likely cause for the parenchymal abnormality observed in the right lower lobe in this patient?

2. Name the term that is used to describe the whorled appearance of the adjacent bronchovascular bundles.

3. What occupational exposure is most closely related to this process?

4. Is rounded atelectasis associated only with asbestos-related pleural disease?

Rounded Atelectasis

1. Rounded atelectasis.

2. The "comet tail sign."

3. Asbestos.

4. No.

Reference

Batra P, Brown K, Hayashi K, Mori M: Rounded atelectasis. *J Thorac Imaging* 11:187-197, 1996.

Cross-Reference

Thoracic Radiology: THE REQUISITES, 2nd ed, pp 211-212.

Comment

Rounded atelectasis refers to a form of peripheral focal atelectasis that develops in patients with pleural disease. Although it is most commonly associated with asbestos-related pleural disease, rounded atelectasis may occur in the setting of chronic pleural thickening or effusion from any etiology.

On chest radiography, it typically appears as a subpleural round or oval, sharply marginated mass that occurs most commonly in the posterior aspect of the lower lobes. The mass usually abuts an area of pleural thickening, which is usually greatest in dimension near the mass. The mass forms acute angles with the adjacent lung parenchyma and is usually separated from the diaphragm by interposed aerated lung.

A characteristic feature of rounded atelectasis is the presence of a curvilinear tail, which has been referred to as the *comet tail sign.* This refers to the presence of crowded bronchi and blood vessels that extend from the lower border of the mass and converge to the adjacent hilum, creating a whorled appearance of the bronchovascular bundle. Signs of volume loss are occasionally evident on chest radiography but are usually minimal. On CT, displacement of the adjacent fissure is frequently observed.

In this case, the CT findings of a focal parenchymal opacity adjacent to an area of pleural thickening with associated volume loss and a comet tail sign are diagnostic of rounded atelectasis. For cases in which the CT findings are equivocal, fine-needle aspiration biopsy is suggested to exclude malignancy because of the high association between lung cancer and asbestos exposure in smokers. PET imaging typically shows no FDG avidity, but low-level uptake has been described in some cases.

Notes

1. Name at least four causes of an upper zone distribution of chronic infiltrative lung disease.

2. Which of these entities are most closely associated with a reticular and nodular pattern on chest radiographs?

3. What is the term used to describe irregular bronchial dilation associated with pulmonary fibrosis?

4. What laboratory test is usually elevated in patients with sarcoidosis?

Sarcoidosis

1. Silicosis, coal worker's pneumoconiosis, sarcoidosis, ankylosing spondylitis, Langerhans cell histiocytosis (LCH), and chronic berylliosis.

2. Sarcoidosis and LCH.

3. Traction bronchiectasis.

4. Angiotensin-converting enzyme (ACE) levels.

Reference

Miller BH, Rosado-de-Christenson ML, McAdams HP, Fishback NF: Thoracic sarcoidosis: radiologic-pathologic correlation. *Radiographics* 15:421-437, 1995.

Cross-Reference

Thoracic Radiology: THE REQUISITES, 2nd ed, pp 188-190.

Comment

The chest radiograph reveals a bilateral upper lung zone distribution of reticular and nodular opacities with associated upper lobe volume loss. The HRCT images in the second and third figures demonstrate irregular linear and small nodular opacities with associated architectural distortion and traction bronchiectasis and bronchiolectasis.

Among the various causes of an upper lung zone distribution of chronic infiltrative lung disease, sarcoidosis is most closely associated with a reticular and nodular pattern. Approximately 20% of sarcoid patients with evidence of interstitial lung disease will develop fibrosis. The fibrosis is usually most pronounced in the apical and posterior portions of the upper lobes and in the superior segments of the lower lobes, as demonstrated in this case. Signs of volume loss and architectural distortion are commonly observed, with masslike opacities and areas of traction bronchiectasis.

Notes

1. What vascular abnormality is evident on this MRI?

2. Name at least two entities that may be associated with an ascending aortic aneurysm.

3. Is this a T1W or a T2W image?

4. What is the difference between a true and a false aneurysm?

C A S E 7 6

Ascending Aortic Aneurysm Secondary to Cystic Medial Necrosis

1. Ascending aortic aneurysm.

2. Cystic medial necrosis (Marfan's and Ehlers-Danlos syndromes), atherosclerosis, and syphilis.

3. T1W (note the bright signal intensity of mediastinal fat).

4. A true aneurysm has an intact aortic wall; a false aneurysm is characterized by a disrupted aortic wall.

Reference

Agarwal PP, Chughtal A, Matzinger F, Karerooni EA: Multidetector CT of thoracic aortic aneurysms. *Radiographics* 29:537-552, 2009.

Cross-Reference

Thoracic Radiology: THE REQUISITES, 2nd ed, pp 358-359.

Comment

The coronal MRI in the figure reveals marked aneurysmal dilation of the ascending aorta. An *aneurysm* is defined as an abnormal dilation of a vessel. With regard to the ascending aorta, there is some variability in diameter with increasing patient age, but a diameter of greater than 4 cm is generally considered abnormal.

Aneurysms may be classified on the basis of the integrity of aorta wall (true vs. false), location, and shape. With regard to shape, *fusiform aneurysms* are characterized by cylindrical dilation of the entire circumference of the aorta, and *saccular aneurysms* are characterized by a focal outpouching of the aorta. Fusiform aneurysms are most commonly associated with atherosclerosis, whereas saccular aneurysms are most often traumatic or infections in etiology.

Ascending aortic aneurysms are less common than descending thoracic aortic aneurysms. Although aneurysmal dilation of the ascending aorta is frequently caused by atherosclerosis, this process usually involves other portions of the aorta as well. *Annuloaortic ectasia* refers to the presence of dilated sinuses of Valsalva with effacement of the sinotubular junction, resulting in a pear-shaped ascending aorta that tapers to a normal-caliber aortic arch. This disorder may be idiopathic or associated with connective tissue disorders such as Ehlers-Danlos and Marfan's syndromes. Syphilis, once a relatively common cause of ascending aortic aneurysms, is now rare.

The major complication of aneurysms is rupture. The risk of rupture is related to the size of the aneurysm. For this reason, elective surgical repair is generally recommended when aneurysms exceed 5 to 6 cm in diameter.

Notes

1. Which pulmonary neoplasm is the most likely cause for this centrally obstructing mass that contains calcification?

2. Are carcinoids benign or malignant neoplasms?

3. Name the nuclear medicine study that can be useful for imaging carcinoid tumors.

4. What percentage of carcinoids demonstrate calcification on CT images?

Carcinoid

1. Carcinoid.

2. Malignant.

3. Octreotide scanning.

4. Approximately 30%.

Reference

Chong S, Lee KS, Chung MJ, et al: Neuroendocrine tumors of the lung: clinical, pathologic, and imaging findings. *Radiographics* 26:41-57, 2006.

Cross-Reference

Thoracic Radiology: THE REQUISITES, 2nd ed, pp 269-270.

Comment

The frontal chest radiograph demonstrates a central, right hilar mass with associated partial atelectasis of the right upper lobe. The CT image demonstrates a partially calcified right hilar mass that obstructs the right upper lobe bronchus. The imaging features are characteristic of a central carcinoid tumor.

Bronchial carcinoid tumors are uncommon neuroendocrine neoplasms that occur centrally (80%) more commonly than peripherally (20%). Affected patients are usually in the third to seventh decade of life and typically present with cough, hemoptysis, and postobstructive pneumonia.

On chest radiographs, carcinoids typically appear as a central, hilar, or perihilar mass that may be associated with postobstructive atelectasis, pneumonia, mucoid impaction, or bronchiectasis. On CT, carcinoids typically demonstrate well-defined margins and slightly lobulated borders. Carcinoids are usually located close to the central bronchi, usually near airway bifurcations. Calcification is observed in approximately 30% of cases on CT but is not usually evident on conventional radiographs. Most lesions demonstrate intense contrast enhancement.

A minority of carcinoids present as a solitary pulmonary nodule (SPN) in the periphery of the lung. Typical carcinoid tumors in the periphery of the lungs usually grow at a slow rate. Atypical carcinoids, which account for 10% of all carcinoids, occur most often in the lung periphery. These lesions are usually large at the time of presentation and grow at a faster rate than typical carcinoids. Although typical carcinoids rarely metastasize, atypical carcinoids exhibit metastases in up to half of patients.

Therapy of carcinoid tumors consists of surgical resection, with a more aggressive surgical approach for atypical lesions. Adjuvant chemotherapy has also been employed with some success in patients with advanced atypical carcinoid tumors. Typical carcinoids have an excellent prognosis, with a 5-year survival of approximately 90%. In contrast, atypical carcinoids are associated with a 5-year survival of approximately 70%.

Because carcinoid tumors have a high number of somatostatin receptors, scintigraphic imaging with the radiolabeled somatostatin analogue octreotide may be helpful for detecting occult tumors. Conversely, PET-FDG imaging is less useful in this setting because of a high rate of false-negative results for typical carcinoid tumors.

Notes

1. Name the syndrome that refers to esophageal perforation due to repeated episodes of vomiting.

2. Name at least three other causes of esophageal perforation.

3. Name two sites of abnormal, extraalveolar air collections that may be associated with esophageal perforation.

4. Are pleural complications of esophageal perforation more commonly left- or right-sided?

Boerhaave's Syndrome

1. Boerhaave's syndrome.

2. Iatrogenic, impacted foreign body, obstructing neoplasm, and trauma.

3. Pneumomediastinum and pneumothorax.

4. Left-sided.

Reference

Giménez A, Franquet T, Erasmus JJ, et al: Thoracic complications of esophageal disorders. *Radiographics* 22:S247-S258, 2002.

Cross-Reference

Thoracic Radiology: THE REQUISITES, 2nd ed, pp 370, 371.

Comment

Esophageal perforation is a common cause of acute mediastinitis and may occur secondary to a variety of mechanisms. *Boerhaave's syndrome* refers to transmural perforation of the distal esophagus that occurs secondary to repeated episodes of vomiting. Rupture typically occurs posteriorly, near the left diaphragmatic crus.

Patients with esophageal perforation typically present with symptoms of fever, leukocytosis, dysphagia, and retrosternal chest pain, which often radiates into the neck. Pneumomediastinum is a frequent chest radiographic finding, as demonstrated in this case (note the presence of an abnormal lucency surrounding the ascending aorta and aortic arch and extending into the soft tissues of the lower neck). Additional chest radiographic findings may include diffuse mediastinal widening, pneumothorax (note the presence of a left hydropneumothorax in the figure), pleural effusion, and empyema. When the diagnosis of esophageal perforation is delayed, additional complications may include mediastinal abscess, esophagopleural fistula, and esophagobronchial fistula.

A diagnosis of suspected esophageal perforation can be confirmed by performing a fluoroscopic examination of the esophagus following the administration of water-soluble contrast medium. Such a study demonstrates extravasation of contrast at the site of perforation, but it may be false-negative in up to 10% of cases. CT may be helpful in cases for which fluoroscopy is nondiagnostic. It may also be helpful to delineate the location and extent of fluid collections in cases that have progressed to mediastinal abscess formation.

It is important to be aware that a delay of more than 24 hours in the diagnosis of this complication is associated with high morbidity and mortality rates. Thus, prompt diagnosis and treatment are critical.

Notes

1. In an HIV-positive patient, what is the most likely cause for these CT findings?

2. What organ system is most commonly involved by this neoplasm?

3. Name the demographic group of HIV-positive patients that is most commonly affected by this neoplasm.

4. Is Kaposi's sarcoma (KS) gallium-avid?

Kaposi's Sarcoma

1. KS.

2. Skin.

3. Homosexual men.

4. No.

Reference
Boiselle PM, Aviram G, Fishman JE: Update on lung disease in AIDS. *Semin Roentgenol* 37:54-71, 2002.

Cross-Reference
Thoracic Radiology: THE REQUISITES, 2nd ed, pp 131, 133.

Comment
KS is the most common AIDS-related neoplasm worldwide, but its prevalence has markedly declined in the Western world owing to widespread use of highly active antiretroviral therapy (HAART). It occurs predominantly, but not exclusively, in homosexual men. KS is a multicentric neoplasm that arises from endothelial cells. It may involve multiple organ systems, including the skin, lymphatics, lungs, and gastrointestinal system. It is associated with human herpesvirus 8, also referred to as *Kaposi's sarcoma herpesvirus.*

The CT image in this case demonstrates characteristic lung parenchymal abnormalities of KS, including a peribronchovascular distribution of consolidation and poorly defined lung nodules. Less commonly observed lung parenchymal findings may include interlobular septal thickening and ground-glass attenuation. The latter is usually observed around the perimeter of lung nodules and masses. Pleural effusions and thoracic lymph node enlargement are relatively common thoracic manifestations of KS and frequently accompany pulmonary parenchymal abnormalities.

Nuclear medicine imaging may be helpful in the assessment of HIV-positive patients with suspected pulmonary KS. Unlike pulmonary infections and lymphoma, KS is not gallium-avid. Thus, in an HIV-positive patient with diffuse parenchymal abnormalities, the absence of increased gallium activity within the lungs can help confirm the diagnosis of KS and exclude a coexisting infection or alternative diagnosis such as lymphoma.

Notes

1. Define a bulla.

2. Define a bleb.

3. Name at least two potential complications of bullae.

4. What is the treatment for symptomatic bullae?

Bulla

1. A bulla is a sharply demarcated airspace measuring more than 1 cm in diameter and possessing a well-defined wall less than 1 mm in thickness.

2. A bleb is a small (less than 1 cm) gas-containing space within the visceral pleura or in the subpleural lung.

3. Pneumothorax, infection, and hemorrhage.

4. Surgical resection (bullectomy).

Reference

Arroliga AC: Lung volume reduction and bullectomy in COPD. In: Rose BD, Ed. *UpToDate*. Waltham, MA, UpToDate, 2009.

Cross-Reference

Thoracic Radiology: THE REQUISITES, 2nd ed, pp 51, 53, 245, 246.

Comment

The chest radiograph and the CT image demonstrate a large bulla within the right upper lobe.

Bullae may develop in association with any type of emphysema, but they are most commonly associated with paraseptal and centrilobular emphysema. However, they are not always associated with diffuse emphysema.

Bullae usually enlarge over months to years, but the growth rate is quite variable. Occasionally, bullae can become quite large and may be focal in distribution. Large bullae may compromise respiratory function. The resulting syndrome has been referred to by various terms, including *bullous emphysema, vanishing lung syndrome,* and *primary bullous disease of the lung.* This entity occurs most often in young men and is characterized by large, progressive upper lobe bullous disease. Although it may occur in nonsmokers, most affected patients are smokers.

CT is the preferred modality for the assessment of patients with suspected bullous emphysema. CT is helpful for delineating the number, size, and location of bullae. It can also assess the degree of compression of underlying normal lung and determine the presence and severity of emphysema in the remaining portion of the lung parenchyma.

In symptomatic patients, surgical resection of bullae can result in marked improvement in pulmonary function. The greatest benefit from surgery is observed in patients with a large bulla (occupying 50% or more of a hemithorax) and a moderate reduction in forced expiratory volume in 1 second (FEV_1). In contrast, patients with severe generalized emphysema tend to do poorly and are thus not ideal candidates for bullectomy.

Notes

1. What lobe(s) is collapsed in the first figure?

2. What lobe(s) is collapsed in the second figure?

3. In a patient with a known extrathoracic primary neoplasm, what is the likely cause for lobar collapse?

4. Name at least three common sites of primary malignancies that are associated with endobronchial metastases.

Right Middle and Lower Lobe Collapse Secondary to Endobronchial Metastases

1. Right lower lobe.

2. Right middle lobe and right lower lobe.

3. Endobronchial metastases.

4. Kidney, melanoma, thyroid, breast, and colon.

Reference

Seo JB, Im JG, Goo JM, et al: Atypical pulmonary metastases: spectrum of radiologic findings. *Radiographics* 21:403-417, 2001.

Cross-Reference

Thoracic Radiology: THE REQUISITES, 2nd ed, pp 31-37.

Comment

The chest radiograph in the first figure demonstrates complete collapse of the right lower lobe. A subsequent radiograph (second figure) performed several weeks later reveals combined collapse of the right middle and lower lobes. In the first figure, note the characteristic triangular opacity in the right retrocardiac region that is bordered by a displaced major fissure. The appearance is similar to that observed in cases of left lower lobe collapse. In the second figure, note the further increase in degree of volume loss, with displacement of minor and major fissures, accompanied by increased opacity that obscures the right hemidiaphragmatic contour. The appearance is typical of combined right middle and lower lobe collapse.

Combined right middle and lower lobe collapse can occur when a tumor obstructs the bronchus intermedius. This combination is much more common than combined right upper and right middle lobe collapse because the bronchi to these lobes are remote from one another. When the latter combination occurs, the appearance is identical to left upper lobe collapse.

In this patient, the combined lobar collapse occurred secondary to endobronchial metastatic disease. Also note the presence of pulmonary metastases, best visualized in the left lung. Endobronchial metastases are uncommon and are found in less than 5% of patients at autopsy. Presenting symptoms may include cough, wheeze, and hemoptysis. Coughing may infrequently result in expectoration of tumor fragments; rarely, this is the first indication of metastatic disease.

Radiographic findings in the setting of partial airway obstruction include oligemia and air trapping. In the setting of complete bronchial obstruction, findings include lobar, segmental, or subsegmental atelectasis and postobstructive pneumonitis. A hilar or central mass may also be evident.

Notes

1. A region-of-interest measurement of this mass demonstrated Hounsfield units consistent with fat attenuation. What are the two most likely diagnoses?

2. How can you explain the spread of this mass into the axilla?

3. Although this mass is predominantly fat attenuation, it contains a few strands of soft tissue attenuation. Does the latter finding exclude the diagnosis of lipoma?

4. What feature of this mass favors a benign diagnosis?

Lipoma

1. Lipoma and liposarcoma.

2. The mass is likely extrapleural in location rather than truly mediastinal and probably spreads over the apex of the lung into the left axilla.

3. No.

4. Pliability/lack of invasiveness.

Reference

Gaerte SC, Meyer CA, Winer-Muram HT, et al: Fat-containing lesions of the chest. *Radiographics* 22:S61-S78, 2002.

Cross-Reference

None.

Comment

The CT image demonstrates a fat attenuation mass that contains several strands of soft tissue attenuation. The mass extends into the left axilla, but there is no invasion of the ribs or vessels.

Lipomas may occur in a variety of locations in the thorax, including the mediastinum, chest wall, extrapleural space, esophagus, heart, airway, and rarely, the lung parenchyma. Although lipomas typically appear as well-marginated lesions characterized by homogeneous fat attenuation, soft tissue elements may be observed. In such cases, it may not be possible to distinguish lipoma from thymolipoma or low-grade liposarcoma. The pliability and lack of invasiveness of lipomas may aid in their differentiation from liposarcomas; for example, lipomas typically drape around adjacent vessels, ribs, and mediastinal structures without invading them. In contrast with lipomas, liposarcomas typically contain a larger soft tissue component, have irregular margins, and frequently invade adjacent mediastinal and chest wall structures. Thus, the presence of well-defined margins and lack of invasiveness favor a diagnosis of lipoma over liposarcoma. The diagnosis of lipoma was confirmed at pathology.

Notes

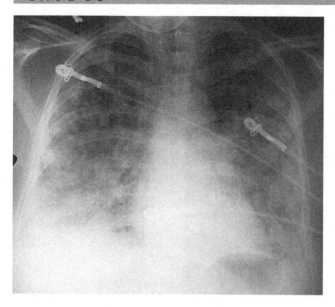

1. Which type of viral pneumonia typically presents with a diffuse distribution of poorly defined lung nodules?

2. What is the approximate overall incidence of pneumonia in patients with chickenpox?

3. Do pregnant women have a higher or lower incidence of varicella pneumonia than the general population?

4. What is the typical radiographic appearance of healed varicella pneumonia?

Varicella-Zoster (Chickenpox)

1. Varicella-zoster (chickenpox).

2. Approximately 15%.

3. Higher.

4. Diffuse, discrete pulmonary calcifications.

Reference

Müller NL, Silva CI: Viruses. In: Müller NL, Silva CI, Eds. *Imaging of the Chest*. Philadelphia, Saunders, 2008, pp 402-404.

Cross-Reference

Thoracic Radiology: THE REQUISITES, 2nd ed, pp 96, 99.

Comment

The chest radiograph demonstrates a diffuse distribution of poorly defined small lung nodules, some of which have coalesced to form areas of consolidation. The appearance is typical of varicella-zoster (chickenpox) pneumonia. Characteristic CT findings (not shown) include 1- to 10-mm nodules diffusely distributed throughout the lungs. Less common findings at CT include nodules with surrounding ground-glass halos, patchy ground-glass opacities, and coalescing nodules.

The varicella-zoster virus is seen in two clinical forms: chickenpox (varicella) and zoster (shingles). Chickenpox represents the primary form of the virus and usually presents as disseminated disease in previously uninfected individuals. Conversely, zoster represents reactivation of a latent virus and typically manifests as a unilateral dermatologic skin eruption. Although either form of the virus may be associated with pneumonia, the majority of cases occur in association with chickenpox.

The overall incidence of pneumonia in adults with chickenpox ranges from 5% to 50%. Predisposing factors include leukemia, lymphoma, immunodeficiency, and pregnancy. Both the incidence and the severity of varicella pneumonia are significantly higher in pregnant women than in the general population.

Acute chickenpox pneumonia is most common in adult patients with severe cutaneous disease. Affected patients typically present 2 or 3 days following the appearance of a skin eruption with symptoms of cough, dyspnea, tachypnea, and pleuritic chest pain.

Acute chickenpox pneumonia is associated with a mortality rate as high as 10%. In patients who survive the infection, clinical improvement usually precedes radiographic clearing by several weeks. A characteristic radiologic finding in patients with healed varicella pneumonia is the presence of diffuse discrete pulmonary calcifications.

Notes

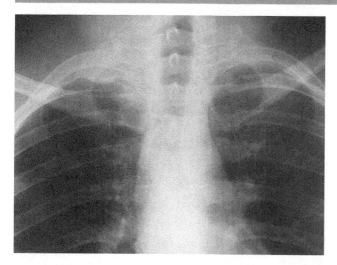

1. Name at least four causes of a unilateral, enlarged apical cap.

2. What is the term used to describe a primary lung cancer that arises at the apex of the lung?

3. Regarding extrapleural apical lesions, are their margins usually smooth or irregular?

4. This patient presented with a palpable right-sided neck mass. Name two possible causes for the enlarged apical cap in this case.

CASE 84

Apical Cap Secondary to Extrapleural Abscess Extending From the Neck

1. Primary lung cancer, lymphoma extending from the neck or mediastinum, extrapleural hematoma related to injury, extrapleural abscess extending from the neck, and radiation fibrosis.

2. Superior sulcus tumor.

3. Smooth.

4. Extrapleural extension of neck abscess and lymphoma.

Reference

McLoud TC, Isler RJ, Novelline RA, et al: The apical cap. *AJR Am J Roentgenol* 137:299-306, 1981.

Cross-Reference

None.

Comment

The term *apical cap* has been used to describe the presence of an opacity located in the extreme apex of the lung on chest radiographs. On chest radiographs of normal, asymptomatic patients, you will often observe the apical cap as an irregular opacity located over the apex of the lung, usually measuring less than 5 mm in diameter. The lower margin is usually sharply marginated but often demonstrates an undulating border. Apical caps are thought to represent the result of nonspecific subpleural scarring and apical pleural thickening, and they are usually of no clinical significance. The prevalence of apical caps increases with age.

A variety of entities may result in an enlarged apical cap. The various causes of a unilateral enlarged cap have been listed in Answer 1. With regard to bilaterally enlarged apical caps, they may be associated with radiation fibrosis (e.g., for Hodgkin's disease), mediastinal lipomatosis, and vascular abnormalities such as coarctation of the aorta.

In this case, the presence of a smoothly marginated enlarged right apical cap is due to extension of a neck abscess into the lung apex. Because of the continuity of the fascial planes of the neck with the thoracic apical region, infectious processes originating in the neck may extend into the area of the lung apex, within the extrapleural space. The apical cap in such cases is smoothly marginated, reflecting the extrapleural location. Lymphoma is an additional important consideration in this case. In patients with lymphoma, an apical cap may be produced by extension of lymphadenopathy from the neck or by enlargement of lymph nodes along the apical pleura.

Notes

1. What is the etiology of the abnormal low-attenuation areas present in both lungs on these HRCT images?

2. What types of emphysema are evident in this case?

3. What type of emphysema is most closely associated with cigarette smoking?

4. What portion of the lungs is most commonly affected by this type of emphysema?

Emphysema

1. Emphysema.

2. Centrilobular and paraseptal.

3. Centrilobular.

4. Upper lobes.

Reference

Kazerooni EA, Whyte RI, Flint A, Martinez FJ: Imaging of emphysema and lung volume reduction surgery. *Radiographics* 17:1023-1036, 1997.

Cross-Reference

Thoracic Radiology: THE REQUISITES, 2nd ed, pp 242-248.

Comment

The HRCT image and magnified view of the left lung demonstrate multiple foci of low attenuation, consistent with emphysema. Note the absence of definable walls for most of the areas of abnormal low attenuation.

Features of both centrilobular and paraseptal emphysema are present. *Centrilobular emphysema* is characterized by multiple small, round foci of abnormally low attenuation, typically without visible walls, that are scattered throughout the lung parenchyma. *Paraseptal emphysema* is characterized by its location within the subpleural regions and adjacent to the interlobar fissures. Foci of paraseptal emphysema often have thin visible walls that correspond to interlobular septa. In this case, paraseptal emphysema is best demonstrated adjacent to the anterior pleural surfaces. When larger than a centimeter in size, foci of paraseptal emphysema and/or confluent areas of centrilobular emphysema, are most appropriately referred to as "bullae."

HRCT of the chest is highly sensitive and specific for the diagnosis of emphysema. It is particularly helpful for assessing the severity and distribution of emphysema in patients who are potential candidates for lung volume reduction surgery (LVRS). LVRS is a procedure that involves the resection of "target areas" of severely emphysematous lung. Such regions contribute little to pulmonary function and negatively alter respiratory mechanics. LVRS usually involves bilateral wedge resection procedures performed via a median sternotomy.

Improved pulmonary function following LVRS is thought to be due to several factors, including improved elastic recoil of the lungs, correction of $\dot{V}/\dot{Q}$ mismatches, and improved mechanics of breathing. Patients are selected for the procedure based on a variety of clinical and imaging parameters. With regard to imaging features, preliminary data suggest that patients with a heterogeneous distribution of emphysema with an upper lobe predominance are most likely to benefit from this procedure.

Notes

1. This patient has a history of lymphoma and is being treated with bleomycin. What is the most likely cause for the interstitial opacities observed in the first and second figures?

2. Approximately what percentage of patients receiving bleomycin develop pulmonary toxicity?

3. Does simultaneous chest radiation therapy increase or decrease the risk of bleomycin pulmonary toxicity?

4. Would you expect this patient's diffusing capacity of carbon monoxide (DLCO) to be increased or decreased?

Bleomycin Drug Toxicity

1. Bleomycin pulmonary toxicity.

2. Approximately 4%.

3. Increase.

4. Decreased.

Reference

Rossi SE, Erasmus JJ, McAdams HP, et al: Pulmonary drug toxicity: radiologic and pathologic manifestations. *Radiographics* 20:1245-1259, 2000.

Cross-Reference

Thoracic Radiology: THE REQUISITES, 2nd ed, pp 236-237.

Comment

The chest radiograph in the first figure reveals the presence of reticular opacities within the peripheral and basilar portions of the lung parenchyma. The CT images in the second and third figures demonstrate thickened septal lines, irregular linear opacities, ground-glass opacities, and several tiny lung nodules in a subpleural and basilar predominance.

Bleomycin is an antitumor agent that is used to treat lymphomas, testicular carcinomas, and certain squamous cell carcinomas. Pulmonary toxicity occurs in approximately 4% of patients and is the principal dose-limiting factor for this agent. Pulmonary fibrosis is the most serious pulmonary complication, but an acute hypersensitivity reaction occurs rarely.

Affected patients typically present with an insidious onset of dyspnea, nonproductive cough, and occasional fever. Pulmonary function tests reveal a decreased DLCO, a sensitive measure for early bleomycin lung injury.

Chest radiographs may be normal or may demonstrate reticular opacities in a basilar and subpleural distribution, similar to those observed in idiopathic pulmonary fibrosis. CT (especially HRCT) is more sensitive that conventional radiographs for detecting interstitial abnormalities and may reveal characteristic findings even when the chest radiograph is normal. Pulmonary nodules are an uncommon manifestation of bleomycin toxicity and usually represent drug-induced COP (cryptogenic organizing pneumonia). Nodules may vary in size from 5 mm to 3 cm and are usually subpleural in distribution.

Early detection is important because prompt discontinuation of bleomycin may result in improved pulmonary function and healing of pulmonary damage in patients with early stages of disease. In patients with more advanced disease, the prognosis is variable. Although some patients respond to steroids, others develop progressive fibrosis that may lead to respiratory failure and death.

Notes

1. In an HIV-positive patient, which fungal infection is most likely to present with pulmonary nodules, pleural effusion, and lymph node enlargement?

2. Are pleural effusions and thoracic lymph node enlargement more commonly observed in immunocompetent or immunosuppressed patients with cryptococcal pulmonary infection?

3. What organ system is most commonly affected by this organism?

4. What other organ systems are commonly involved in disseminated cryptococcal infection?

AIDS Cryptococcal Infection

1. Cryptococcus.

2. Immunosuppressed.

3. Central nervous system (meningitis).

4. Bone and skin.

Reference

Avriam G, Fishman JE, Boiselle PM: Thoracic infections in human immunodeficiency virus/acquired immune deficiency syndrome. *Semin Roentgenol* 42:23-36, 2007.

Cross-Reference

Thoracic Radiology: THE REQUISITES, 2nd ed, p 128.

Comment

The CT images in this case demonstrate several small pulmonary nodules with associated left hilar and subcarinal lymph node enlargement and a small left pleural effusion. There are a variety of causes of lung nodules in patients with AIDS, including infectious etiologies (fungal, mycobacterial, septic infarcts) and neoplasms (KS, lymphoma).

Prior to the AIDS epidemic and the advent of immunosuppressive therapies, most cryptococcal infections occurred in immunocompetent hosts. It is estimated that approximately 70% of such infections now occur in immunosuppressed patients. In immunocompetent hosts, the infection is usually localized to the lung. In contrast, in immunosuppressed patients, dissemination to the central nervous system and skin is common. Pulmonary symptoms are uncommon in both groups. However, immunosuppressed patients with disseminated disease frequently present with symptoms related to the central nervous system or skeletal system.

A variety of imaging features are associated with this infection. Common manifestations in both immunosuppressed and immunocompetent hosts include solitary or multiple pulmonary nodules and masses and segmental or lobar consolidation. Other features, including diffuse reticulonodular opacities, cavitating nodules or masses, pleural effusion, and mediastinal and hilar lymph node enlargement, are more commonly observed in immunosuppressed patients than in normal hosts.

Notes

1. Transthoracic biopsy of the lung mass shown in the figures revealed NSCLC. Is the presence of an enlarged aortopulmonary window lymph node sufficient proof of metastatic nodal disease?

2. Based on the TNM classification system for NSCLC, if this node is proved malignant, what would be the N status of the patient?

3. Does this nodal status preclude surgical resection?

4. What is the significance of contralateral nodal disease in patients with NSCLC?

C A S E 8 8

Lung Cancer With N2 Nodal Disease

1. No.

2. N2.

3. No.

4. It precludes surgical resection.

References

Sharma A, Fidias P, Hayman LA, et al: Patterns of lymph-adenopathy in thoracic malignancies. *Radiographics* 24:419-434, 2004.

Kligerman S, Abbott G: A radiologic review of the new TNM classification for lung cancer. *AJR Am J Roentgenol* 194:562-573, 2010.

Cross-Reference

Thoracic Radiology: THE REQUISITES, 2nd ed, pp 263-268.

Comment

In patients with NSCLC, the nodal status provides important information for determining prognosis and planning appropriate therapy. Although no changes are planned for the N designation in the seventh edition of the TNM classification system, a new nodal chart has been created that places lymph nodes into seven specific zones: supraclavicular, upper, aorticopulmonary, subcarinal, lower, hilar-interlobar, and peripheral.

According to the TNM classification system, nodal involvement is graded from N0 to N3 as follows:

N0 = no demonstrable metastases to regional lymph nodes.

N1 = metastasis to lymph nodes in the ipsilateral peripheral, or hilar-interlobar regions.

N2 = metastasis to ipsilateral mediastinal nodes (upper, aorticopulmonary, lower or subcarinal).

N3 = metastasis to any supraclavicular nodes, or to contralateral mediastinal (upper, aorticopulmonary, lower), hilar-interlobar, or peripheral regions.

CT and MRI play an important but limited role in the assessment of nodal status in patients with bronchogenic carcinoma. These imaging modalities rely primarily on anatomic features of lymph nodes, most notably lymph node size (short axis greater than 1 cm diameter is generally considered abnormal). This strategy is associated with sensitivities in the range of 60% to 79% and specificities in the range of 60% to 80%. Thus, for staging purposes, enlarged nodes must be evaluated by biopsy. The primary role of these modalities is to identify the location of enlarged nodes. This information allows appropriate biopsy procedures to be planned.

In recent years, FDG-PET imaging has been shown to be superior to CT and MRI in the assessment of mediastinal lymph nodes. This technique relies on physiologic (glucose metabolism) rather than anatomic features to identify abnormal lymph nodes. Thus, it has the potential to identify neoplastic involvement within small nodes and to differentiate enlarged, hyperplastic nodes from neoplastic nodes.

Notes

1. What is the most common cause of superior vena cava (SVC) syndrome?

2. Name at least one common benign cause of SVC syndrome.

3. Name at least two mechanisms by which the SVC may become obstructed.

4. What are the typical clinical symptoms of a patient with SVC obstruction?

SVC Syndrome

1. Malignancy—lung cancer.

2. Long-term intravenous devices; fibrosing mediastinitis.

3. Extrinsic compression, direct invasion, and intraluminal thrombus.

4. Edema of the face, neck, upper extremities, and thorax; headache; visual disturbances; and reduced level of consciousness.

Reference

Eran S, Karaman A, Okur A: The superior vena cava syndrome caused by malignant disease: imaging with multidetector row CT. *Eur J Radiol* 59:93-103, 2006.

Cross-Reference

Thoracic Radiology: THE REQUISITES, 2nd ed, p 262.

Comment

The SVC syndrome is caused by obstruction of the SVC by either external compression, intraluminal thrombosis, neoplastic infiltration, or a combination of these processes. The vast majority of cases occur secondary to a neoplastic process, most commonly bronchogenic carcinoma (especially small cell carcinoma). Lymphoma and metastatic carcinoma are additional malignant causes. There are a variety of benign etiologies, including long-term intravenous devices (e.g., Hickman catheters and permanent pacemakers) and fibrosing mediastinitis (e.g., histoplasmosis).

Chest radiographs frequently demonstrate a mass in the right paratracheal region, which may be accompanied by distention of the azygos vein. In the setting of fibrosing mediastinitis, the right paratracheal mass is frequently calcified. In patients who develop thrombosis of the SVC owing to an indwelling catheter, lateral displacement of the catheter may be seen. The diagnosis of SVC obstruction can be confirmed by CT or MRI. On CT, the diagnosis is based on decreased or absent contrast opacification of the SVC in conjunction with opacification of collateral vessels. Both findings are necessary to make a reliable diagnosis. Contrast-enhanced MDCT with multiplanar reformation and three-dimensional reconstructions is highly accurate at detecting the presence and level of SVC obstruction. It is also valuable for helping to determine the cause of obstruction and for delineating the collateral venous circulation.

When you observe collateral venous vessels, you should always search for a central venous obstruction.

Notes

1. What is the term used to describe the presence of periosteal reaction in association with pulmonary disease?

2. Are benign or malignant disorders more commonly associated with this process?

3. When this process occurs in association with a pulmonary malignancy, what is the usual response of the periosteal reaction following pulmonary neoplasm resection?

4. Is this skeletal process typically symptomatic?

Hypertrophic Pulmonary Osteoarthropathy

1. Hypertrophic pulmonary osteoarthropathy (HPOA).

2. Malignant.

3. Resolution.

4. Yes—it is usually associated with pain, swelling, and stiffness.

Reference

Love C, Din AS, Tomas MB, et al: Radionuclide bone imaging: an illustrative review. *Radiographics* 23:341-358, 2003.

Cross-Reference

Thoracic Radiology: THE REQUISITES, 2nd ed, pp 256-257.

Comment

The radiographs of the right ankle shown in the first figure reveal the presence of smoothly marginated periosteal reaction along the shafts of the distal tibia and fibula. A similar appearance was present in radiographs of the remaining extremities (not shown).

The term *HPOA* is used to describe the association between this skeletal condition and visceral disease within an organ supplied by the vagal or glossopharyngeal nerves. Although there are a variety of pulmonary and extrapulmonary causes of this condition, malignant pulmonary neoplasms account for the vast majority (90%) of cases. Because of this strong association, you should always recommend that a patient with evidence of HPOA undergo a chest radiograph to assess for pulmonary neoplasm or other causes of pulmonary disease. Note the large central neoplasm on the chest radiograph of this patient in the second figure. Common nonneoplastic pulmonary conditions include cystic fibrosis and idiopathic pulmonary fibrosis. Localized fibrous lesions of the pleura are also frequently associated with this condition.

The underlying mechanism of this condition is poorly understood, but it is believed to be due to an osteogenic effect exerted by a cytokine. Vascular endothelial growth factor (VEGF) has recently been suggested as a possible cytokine for inciting this reaction. Interestingly, following resection of an associated thoracic malignancy, HPOA usually disappears.

Notes

1. Does this patient have an acute pulmonary embolus?

2. What is the cause of the focal decrease in caliber of the descending left pulmonary artery?

3. In patients with sarcoidosis, how frequently do enlarged nodes result in compression of pulmonary arteries?

4. What vascular structure appears abnormally dilated in the first figure?

Extrinsic Compression of Pulmonary Arteries (Sarcoid)

1. No.

2. Extrinsic compression by adjacent nodal tissue.

3. Rarely.

4. Main pulmonary artery.

Reference

Hennebicque AS, Nunes H, Brillet PY, et al: CT findings in severe thoracic sarcoidosis. *Eur Radiol* 15:23-30, 2005.

Cross-Reference

Thoracic Radiology: THE REQUISITES, 2nd ed, pp 334, 335.

Comment

The CT pulmonary angiogram images in the first (axial) and second (coronal reformation) figures reveal extrinsic narrowing of the descending left pulmonary artery and superior segment right lower lobe pulmonary artery by adjacent nodal tissue.

This patient has a history of sarcoidosis. Occasionally, enlarged nodes in patients with sarcoidosis are sufficiently large to compress the bronchi. Rarely, enlarged nodes may result in narrowing of pulmonary arteries, as demonstrated in this case. Massively enlarged right paratracheal nodes have been reported to obstruct the superior vena cava.

In patients with sarcoidosis, pulmonary arterial hypertension is usually secondary to end-stage pulmonary fibrosis. However, it may rarely occur secondary to extrinsic compression of major pulmonary arteries by enlarged lymph nodes or by compression and obliteration of small arterioles by adjacent granulomas.

When interpreting CT pulmonary angiograms, it is important to distinguish pulmonary emboli from extrinsic abnormalities such as lymph nodes. Note the absence of intrinsic filling defects within the pulmonary vasculature in this case. One additional distinguishing feature is the size of the pulmonary arteries. In the setting of an acute pulmonary embolus, the affected vessel is often dilated. In contrast, when extrinsically compressed, the vessel will be abnormally narrowed. Extrinsic compression may be more difficult to distinguish from chronic pulmonary emboli, which result in mural rather than central pulmonary artery filling defects. Recognition that the abnormal soft tissue attenuation material is extrinsic rather than intrinsic to the vessel allows one to exclude chronic pulmonary embolus. Although this distinction can usually be made readily on conventional axial images (as is true in this case), supplemental multiplanar reformatted images are helpful for difficult cases.

Notes

1. This patient has a history of hemophilia. What is the likely cause for this posterior chest wall mass?

2. What does the high-attenuation component of the mass represent on this unenhanced CT scan study?

3. Name at least two potential complications of intramuscular hemorrhage.

4. How is hemophilia genetically transmitted?

Chest Wall Hematoma in Hemophilia

1. Hematoma.

2. Acute hemorrhage.

3. Joint contractures, ischemic myopathy, neuropathy, pressure necrosis of adjacent bone, and pseudotumor formation.

4. X-linked recessive; thus, hemophilia is transmitted by females but primarily affects males.

Reference
Park JS, Ryu KN: Hemophilic pseudotumor involving the musculoskeletal system: spectrum of radiologic findings. *AJR Am J Roentgenol* 183:55-61, 2004.

Cross-Reference
None.

Comment
The CT images reveal a large, well-marginated, heterogeneous posterior chest wall mass with its epicenter in the left paraspinal musculature. The high attenuation of this mass on an unenhanced CT is consistent with the diagnosis of acute intramuscular hematoma, a known complication of hemophilia.

Hemophilia refers to a disorder characterized by a coagulation defect caused by a deficiency of clotting factor. Repetitive bleeding into the musculoskeletal system is the most common complication of this condition. The joint spaces are the most common site of spontaneous bleeding. Hemarthrosis is frequently complicated by arthritis. The soft tissues, particularly large muscle groups, are also a relatively common site of hemorrhage. The most commonly affected muscle groups are the iliopsoas, quadriceps, and gastrocnemius. If bleeding into the hematoma is replaced by fibrous tissue, a permanent contracture may develop. Encapsulation of a hematoma may result in the formation of a pseudotumor.

Cross-sectional imaging studies can be helpful for identifying the site and extent of intramuscular hematomas in patients with hemophilia. Because of its relative low cost and lack of ionizing radiation, ultrasonography is usually the preferred modality for this purpose. In patients with large hematomas, CT and MRI are occasionally helpful for determining the extent of hemorrhage, estimating the age of hemorrhage, and demonstrating the effect of the hemorrhage on adjacent organs.

Notes

A

B

1. What feature suggests a benign, nonaggressive etiology of this rib lesion?

2. Name at least two likely causes of this rib lesion.

3. Name an entity that may be associated with chronic infiltrative lung disease and lucent bone lesions.

4. Name at least three primary neoplasms that are frequently associated with lytic bone metastases.

Enchondroma

1. Well-circumscribed, sclerotic margins.

2. Fibrous dysplasia, aneurysmal bone cyst, enchondroma, nonossifying fibroma, and Langerhans cell histiocytosis (LCH).

3. LCH (although pulmonary involvement is usually not accompanied by bone lesions).

4. Lung, breast (lytic or blastic), kidney, and thyroid.

Reference

Guttentag AR, Salwen JK: Keep your eyes on the ribs: the spectrum of normal variants and diseases that involve the ribs. *Radiographics* 19:1125-1142, 1999.

Cross-Reference

None.

Comment

The coned-down chest radiograph in the first figure and the coned-down rib radiograph in the second figure reveal a well-circumscribed, expansile, lucent lesion in the left fourth anterior rib with sclerotic margins. The well-defined, sclerotic margins suggest a nonaggressive rather than an aggressive (e.g., neoplasm, infection) etiology. In contrast, aggressive lucent lesions are typically characterized by poorly defined margins.

There are a variety of causes of benign lucent rib lesions. Careful inspection of this lesion reveals subtle foci of calcification within the lucent center of this lesion. This finding suggests a cartilaginous lesion such as enchondroma. In approximately 50% of cases, such lesions demonstrate calcification, which is usually manifested by punctate foci or rings and arcs of calcification. Enchondromas are asymptomatic unless complicated by pathologic fracture or rare malignant degeneration to chondrosarcoma. The latter should be suspected when a patient with an enchondroma presents with pain in the absence of trauma.

The most common nonneoplastic lesion of the thoracic skeleton is fibrous dysplasia. In patients with this disorder, the rib lesion is usually monostotic and asymptomatic. However, patients may present with symptoms if the lesion is complicated by pathologic fracture. In cases of polyostotic fibrous dysplasia, there is usually a unilateral predominance. Rarely, the degree of thoracic involvement is sufficient to result in progressive restrictive lung disease, pulmonary hypertension, and cor pulmonale. *McCune-Albright syndrome* refers to the presence of polyostotic fibrous dysplasia accompanied by café au lait skin lesions and precocious puberty.

Notes

1. What structure is delineated between the *arrows* on the lateral chest radiograph in the second figure?

2. Is this abnormally widened?

3. What do the lucencies on either side of this structure represent?

4. What descriptor is used to characterize the typical appearance of the cardiac contour in the setting of a pericardial effusion?

C A S E 9 4

Pericardial Effusion

1. Pericardium.

2. Yes—it is widened by the presence of pericardial effusion.

3. Fat.

4. Water bottle or flask shape.

Reference
Cardiac Radiology: THE REQUISITES, pp 265-270.

Cross-Reference
None.

Comment
The chest radiograph in the first figure demonstrates an enlarged cardiac contour, with a globular configuration. The lateral radiograph in the second figure demonstrates a positive *epicardial fat pad sign (EFPS),* also referred to as the *double-lucency sign.* This sign refers to widening (greater than 4 mm) of the soft tissue opacity of the pericardium between the lucent stripes *(arrows)* that represent fat located anterior and posterior (epicardial) to the pericardium. These lucent stripes are demarcated by *paired arrows* on the coned-down image of the lateral chest radiograph in the third figure. The EFPS has a relatively low sensitivity but a high specificity for detecting pericardial effusion.

Chest radiography is associated with a relatively poor sensitivity for detecting pericardial effusions. It has been estimated that approximately 200 ml of pericardial fluid must be present to reliably make the diagnosis radiographically. In contrast, echocardiography is highly sensitive for detecting pericardial effusion and is the study of choice for screening patients with suspected pericardial effusion. MRI may be helpful for characterizing complex pericardial fluid collections.

There are a variety of causes of pericardial effusion, including infection, trauma, radiation therapy, collagen vascular diseases, metabolic disorders, and neoplasms. The most common cause is myocardial infarction with left ventricular failure. *Dressler's syndrome* refers to the development of pericardial and pleural effusions 2 to 10 weeks following myocardial infarction. Such effusions can be hemorrhagic, particularly in patients who have received anticoagulation therapy. The patient in this case developed pericardial and pleural effusions following myocardial infarction.

Notes

1. Is this a case of cystic lung disease or bronchiectasis?

2. How can you make this distinction?

3. What are the three classifications of bronchiectasis (Reid classification)?

4. Name at least three congenital or developmental disorders associated with bronchiectasis.

Bronchiectasis

1. Bronchiectasis.

2. Many of the cystic spaces are connected, several run parallel to adjacent vessels ("signet ring sign"), and several have air-fluid levels.

3. Cylindrical, varicose, and cystic (saccular).

4. Williams-Campbell syndrome, cystic fibrosis, primary hypogammaglobulinemia, "yellow nail" syndrome, immotile cilia syndrome (Kartagener's syndrome), Young's syndrome, and Mounier-Kuhn syndrome.

Reference

Javidan-Nejad C, Bhalla S: Bronchiectasis. *Radiol Clin North Am* 47:289-306, 2009.

Cross-Reference

Thoracic Radiology: THE REQUISITES, 2nd ed, pp 314-318.

Comment

The term *bronchiectasis* refers to abnormal, irreversible dilation of the bronchi. The definitive pathologic description of bronchiectasis was reported by Reid and is based on the morphology of the bronchi and the number of bronchial subdivisions that are present. In *cylindrical bronchiectasis,* the bronchi are minimally dilated and have a straight, regular contour. The average number of bronchial subdivisions from the hilum to the lung periphery is 16 (17 to 20 is normal). In *varicose bronchiectasis,* the bronchi demonstrate a beaded appearance with sequential dilation and constriction. The average number of bronchial divisions is 8. In *cystic bronchiectasis,* the bronchi have a ballooned appearance. The average number of bronchial divisions is only 4.

You can distinguish bronchiectasis from cystic lung disease by using the following criteria. First, when dilated bronchi course perpendicular to the scanning plane, you will always see a pulmonary artery running adjacent to it (signet ring sign). In contrast, true lung cysts, such as those associated with LAM, are located randomly in the lung parenchyma. Second, when dilated bronchi course parallel to the scanning plane, you will observe that the cystic spaces connect with one another. This feature is nicely demonstrated in this case. Finally, cystic bronchiectasis is often associated with fluid levels, a finding that is not generally observed in cystic lung disease.

Notes

1. Name the structure that is likely responsible for displacement of the azygoesophageal contour *(arrows)* in this patient.

2. Why does this appear as a stripe rather than an interface?

3. What imaging study would be most helpful for further evaluation of this finding?

4. Name at least two causes of thoracic esophageal dysmotility.

Esophageal Dysmotility (Achalasia)

1. Esophagus.

2. The esophagus is distended with air.

3. Barium swallow.

4. Progressive systemic sclerosis (scleroderma), achalasia, Chagas' disease, systemic diseases (e.g., amyloidosis), and drugs (e.g., anticholinergics).

Reference

Whitten CR, Khan S, Munneke GJ, Grubnic S: A diagnostic approach to mediastinal abnormalities. *Radiographics* 27:657-671, 2007.

Cross-Reference

Thoracic Radiology: THE REQUISITES, 2nd ed, pp 364-365, 366.

Comment

The azygoesophageal interface is produced by the juxtaposition of aerated lung in the right lower lobe and the soft tissue opacity of the right lateral margin of the azygos vein and/or esophagus. On normal chest radiographs, you will observe the azygoesophageal interface beginning at the level of the azygos arch and extending inferiorly to the level of the diaphragm. It normally produces a concave slope as it curves slightly toward the left. Abnormalities of either the azygos vein (e.g., azygos continuation of the inferior vena cava) or the esophagus (e.g., achalasia) may result in rightward displacement of this interface. Subcarinal masses such as bronchogenic cysts and lymph node enlargement may also result in focal rightward displacement of the azygoesophageal interface, usually producing a rightward convexity in the subcarinal region.

The chest radiograph reveals diffuse, rightward displacement of the azygoesophageal contour, which appears as a stripe rather than an interface. When the azygoesophageal contour is displaced by an air-filled, distended esophagus, you will observe a stripe rather than an interface. This patient has a history of achalasia. In most patients with this disorder, the esophagus contains a large amount of retained secretions. Therefore, you will usually see a displaced azygoesophageal interface rather than a stripe. Retained secretions may also result in a discrete air-fluid level within the distended esophagus.

Notes

1. This patient reports recent travel to the southwestern United States. What is the most likely infectious etiology of this cavity?

2. Where else is this organism endemic?

3. Are cavities associated with the initial pneumonic form or the chronic form of this infection?

4. What is the typical pattern associated with disseminated coccidioidomycosis infection?

CASE 97

Cavity Due to Coccidioidomycosis

1. Coccidioidomycosis.

2. Central and South America and northern Mexico.

3. Chronic.

4. Multiple, small nodules.

Reference
Lindell RM, Hartman TE: Fungal infections. In: Müller NL, Silva CI, Eds. *Imaging of the Chest*, Philadelphia, Saunders, 2008, pp 362-365.

Cross-Reference
Thoracic Radiology: THE REQUISITES, 2nd ed, p 110.

Comment
Coccidioidomycosis infection is caused by inhalation of infected spores of *Coccidioides immitis*, a soil inhabitant that is endemic to desert areas. Although most individuals are asymptomatic following exposure, some will experience a mild, flulike illness.

Radiographic findings vary depending on the stage of infection. Following initial inhalation of the spores, there is a local pneumonic response, which is characterized radiographically as an area of consolidation. Such consolidation usually involves less than an entire lobe, is often located in the lower lobes, and usually resolves spontaneously without therapy.

Chronic pulmonary coccidioidomycosis is characterized radiographically by solitary or multiple pulmonary nodules and cavities. Such cavities, as demonstrated in this case, may have variable wall thickness and are usually radiologically indistinguishable from other causes of cavitary lesions. In a minority (10% to 15%) of cases, coccidioidomycosis is associated with characteristic thin-walled ("grapeskin") cavities. Such cavities may rapidly change in size, presumably due to a check-valve communication with the bronchial tree.

Disseminated coccidioidomycosis is rare; it presents radiographically as multiple nodules. The nodules usually range in size from 5 mm to 1 cm in diameter, but smaller miliary nodules may be observed in some cases. The course of disseminated coccidioidomycosis is variable: it may be chronic and insidious or rapidly fatal. The latter usually occurs in patients who are immunocompromised.

Similar to other infections, coccidiomycosis may cause a false-positive result on FDG-PET studies. This may occur in the acute or chronic phase of infection.

Notes

1. This patient's pulmonary venous wedge pressure was elevated. What is the most likely cause for these chest HRCT findings?

2. What chest radiographic finding correlates with the HRCT finding of thickened interlobular septa?

3. Define ground-glass opacity.

4. Name two technical features that are necessary components of HRCT imaging.

Hydrostatic Pulmonary Edema

1. Hydrostatic pulmonary edema.

2. Kerley (septal) lines.

3. Hazy increased opacity of lungs with preservation of bronchial and vascular margin visibility.

4. Thin collimation (1- to 2-mm) and high spatial frequency reconstruction algorithm.

Reference

Storto ML, Kee ST, Golden JA, Webb WR: Hydrostatic pulmonary edema: high-resolution CT findings. *AJR Am J Roentgenol* 165:817-820, 1995.

Cross-Reference

Thoracic Radiology: THE REQUISITES, 2nd ed, pp 330-332.

Comment

Although a diagnosis of congestive heart failure is usually made on the basis of typical clinical and radiographic findings, occasionally patients with unsuspected congestive heart failure are imaged with chest HRCT in search of a cause of dyspnea. Hydrostatic edema is also an occasional incidental finding in patients who are being scanned for other purposes. Thus, it is important to be aware of the typical HRCT features of hydrostatic edema.

On HRCT of patients with hydrostatic edema, you may observe a combination of ground-glass opacity, smoothly thickened septal lines, peribronchovascular interstitial thickening, increased vascular caliber, and thickened fissures. Small pleural effusions, often right-sided, are also frequently observed. There is an absence of signs of fibrosis such as honeycombing, traction bronchiectasis, and architectural distortion. Interestingly, patients with acute congestive heart failure have also been reported to demonstrate occasionally enlarged mediastinal lymph nodes and haziness of the mediastinal fat.

Correlation between imaging findings and clinical data is usually sufficient to confirm the diagnosis. When the diagnosis is in doubt clinically, a follow-up study after diuresis can occasionally be helpful to confirm resolution of abnormalities and to exclude chronic infiltrative lung disease.

Notes

A

B

1. In this patient with a history of breast cancer, what is the most likely cause for the lobulated retrosternal opacity seen on the lateral chest radiograph in the second figure?

2. What other neoplastic process commonly involves this nodal group?

3. Does a normal chest radiograph exclude enlarged nodes at this site?

4. Name the most common site of enlarged nodes in patients with breast cancer.

Internal Mammary Lymph Node Enlargement

1. Enlarged internal mammary lymph nodes.

2. Lymphoma.

3. No.

4. Axilla.

Reference

Sharma A, Fidias P, Hayman LA, et al: Patterns of lymph-adenopathy in thoracic malignancies. *Radiographics* 24:419-434, 2004.

Cross-Reference

Thoracic Radiology: THE REQUISITES, 2nd ed, pp 373-374.

Comment

The serial lateral chest radiographs reveal interval development of a lobulated opacity in the retrosternal region. In a patient with a history of breast cancer, the most likely etiology is enlarged internal mammary lymph nodes, a common site of metastatic disease in such patients. The lymphatics that drain the medial portion of the breasts enter into the internal mammary lymph nodes. Involvement of internal mammary lymph nodes has prognostic significance and influences therapy decisions.

Enlarged internal mammary nodes are generally visible on chest radiographs only when they are considerably enlarged. On a posteroanterior (PA) chest radiograph of a patient with enlarged internal mammary nodes, you may observe a focal parasternal opacity, which is usually seen at the level of the first three intercostal spaces and less frequently at the fourth or fifth level. On a lateral radiograph, you may observe a lobulated retrosternal opacity, as demonstrated in this case. Most often, the opacity is observed at a more superior level than is shown in this case.

A lobulated retrosternal opacity may also be observed in patients with dilated internal mammary vessels. For example, coarctation of the aorta is associated with collateral internal mammary arteries and SVC obstruction is associated with collateral internal mammary veins. The former is associated with a characteristic appearance of the aorta and evidence of rib notching, and the latter is usually associated with a large mass in the right paratracheal region.

Notes

1. The figures are CT images of two different patients undergoing transthoracic needle biopsy (TTNB) procedures. Which patient is least likely to experience a pneumothorax from this procedure? Why?

2. What is the sensitivity of TTNB for malignant nodules?

3. Name at least three complications of TTNB.

4. How can you improve the yield of TTNB for diagnosing benign lesions?

CT-guided TTNB Procedure

1. The patient in the first figure, because the needle does not traverse aerated lung.

2. Greater than 90%.

3. Pneumothorax (20% to 30%); chest tube (5% to 15%); hemoptysis (1% to 10%); seeding of biopsy track; and air embolism.

4. Use a cutting core biopsy needle that provides a histologic specimen.

Reference

Boiselle PM, Shepard JA, Mark EJ, et al: Routine addition of an automated biopsy device to fine-needle aspiration of the lung: a prospective assessment. *AJR Am J Roentgenol* 169:661-666, 1997.

Cross-Reference

Thoracic Radiology: THE REQUISITES, 2nd ed, pp 400-406.

Comment

The CT images demonstrate TTNB procedures of two separate patients. Note that the peripheral mass in the first figure does not require the biopsy needle to traverse aerated lung. Such lesions are associated with a very low pneumothorax rate.

With regard to planning a TTNB procedure, you should first obtain a prebiopsy CT scan. The shortest, most vertical route should be chosen, and the path of the needle should avoid interlobar fissures, pulmonary vessels, bullae, and areas of severe emphysema.

TTNB is a relatively safe and accurate procedure for obtaining biopsy specimens of lung nodules and masses. The sensitivity for malignant nodules is greater than 90%, and the accuracy for differentiating among various cell types of lung cancer is approximately 80%. A major limitation of TTNB using fine-needle aspiration is a relatively low sensitivity (10% to 40%) for making a specific benign diagnosis. However, this ability can be significantly improved by using core needle biopsy devices. Such devices provide histologic specimens that improve the accuracy of diagnosing benign entities such as granulomas, hamartomas, and organizing pneumonia.

It is important to remember that a negative biopsy for malignancy is not diagnostic unless a specific benign diagnosis has been rendered. Indeed, about 30% of nonspecific negative biopsies prove to represent malignancy. Thus, when you receive a nonspecific negative biopsy, you should consider repeating the biopsy with a core biopsy device. A core biopsy device is also recommended for biopsy of lesions with a suspected diagnosis of lymphoma in order to provide sufficient tissue for classification of lymphoma.

Notes

1. Name four disease entities associated with mucoid impaction and mucocele formation.

2. Name six congenital conditions that affect the bronchi.

3. Which anatomic structures enable collateral air drift to occur in the lungs?

4. Name four possible etiologies of a tubular opacity on imaging studies.

Bronchial Atresia

1. Allergic bronchopulmonary aspergillosis (ABPA), obstructing endobronchial tumor, congenital bronchial atresia (CBA), cystic fibrosis.

2. Bronchial (pulmonary) isomerism syndrome, bronchial atresia, congenital bronchiectasis (e.g., cystic fibrosis, Williams-Campbell syndrome), supernumerary bronchus, pig bronchus, cardiac bronchus.

3. Interalveolar pores of Kohn and the canals of Lambert.

4. AVM, partial anomalous pulmonary venous return (PAPVR), pulmonary varix, mucoid impaction.

Reference

Kinsella D, Sissons G, Williams MP: The radiological imaging of bronchial atresia. *Br J Radiol* 65:681-685, 1992.

Cross-Reference

Thoracic Radiology: THE REQUISITES, 2nd ed, pp 60-63.

Comment

CBA is a rare and benign condition characterized by focal atresia of a segmental, subsegmental, or lobar bronchus. The airways distal to the point of atresia are normal and form mucus, but the obstruction to proximal drainage causes accumulation of mucus distal to the point of atresia with resultant mucoid impaction and formation of a mucocele. An important associated feature is hyperinflation of the distal lung parenchyma through collateral air drift. CBA manifests radiologically as a round, ovoid, or branching structure associated with distal hyperinflation, but may be overlooked on the chest radiograph. Although its imaging features are characteristic, CBA is frequently misdiagnosed, often mistaken for an AVM. Because most cases of CBA do not require surgical resection, recognition of its characteristic imaging features is essential for conservative patient management.

The differential diagnosis of CBA includes other causes of mucoid impaction including ABPA, benign and malignant endobronchial tumors (carcinoid, lung cancer), cystic bronchiectasis related to previous pneumonia, and tuberculous bronchostenosis.

Notes

1. Name three diseases that may manifest on CT as centrilobular ground-glass nodules.

2. What anatomic structures are located in the central core of the secondary pulmonary lobule?

3. Name seven pulmonary diseases associated with cigarette smoking.

4. Which type of immunologic reaction is associated with hypersensitivity pneumonitis?

Hypersensitivity Pneumonitis

1. Subacute hypersensitivity pneumonitis (HP), respiratory bronchiolitis, respiratory bronchiolitis–interstitial lung disease (RB-ILD), PCP, pulmonary LCH.

2. Lobular bronchiole, pulmonary artery, and associated peribronchovascular lymphatics.

3. Emphysema, lung cancer, respiratory bronchiolitis, RB-ILD, desquamative interstitial pneumonia (DIP), PLCH, chronic bronchitis.

4. Type IV.

Reference

Kim KI, Kim CW, Lee MK, et al: Imaging of occupational lung disease. *Radiographics* 21:1371-1391, 2001.

Cross-Reference

Thoracic Radiology: THE REQUISITES, 2nd ed, pp 230-233.

Comment

The presence of centrilobular ground-glass nodules on CT/HRCT should prompt consideration of the diagnosis of subacute HP. Affected patients typically present with dyspnea and chronic cough, and the clinical picture may be confused with other forms of interstitial lung disease. Often, the radiologist is the first member of the health care team to suggest the possibility of HP, and the clinical team may then investigate the patient's environmental and occupation exposures to seek a causative antigen. Differential diagnostic considerations for centrilobular ground-glass nodules should include respiratory bronchiolitis, a disease that affects cigarette smokers, and in the proper clinical setting, atypical infection, including PCP. Centrilobular nodules in subacute HP may be of solid (soft tissue) and/or ground-glass attenuation and may be associated with patchy areas of ground-glass attenuation. The findings tend to predominate in the upper lung zones, and air trapping may be present on expiratory CT imaging. Treatment of subacute HP consists of removing the offending antigen from the patient's environment. Chronic forms may require treatment with corticosteroids.

Notes

1. What is the recommended follow-up (Fleischner Society guidelines) to evaluate this 4-mm solid nodule incidentally detected in a 48-year-old man with a 30-pack-year history of cigarette smoking?

2. How would the follow-up recommendations differ if the nodule were of ground-glass opacity?

3. What is the likelihood that an SPN larger than 20 mm is malignant?

4. What do the Fleischner Society guidelines recommend if a 20-mm nodule is detected in a patient with known underlying malignant disease?

Solitary Pulmonary Nodule (SPN), 4 mm

1. CT follow-up at 12 months. If unchanged and of solid (soft tissue) attenuation, no further follow-up is necessary.

2. Nonsolid (ground-glass) or partly solid nodules may require longer follow-up to exclude an indolent adenocarcinoma.

3. 50%.

4. The Fleischner guidelines do not apply to patients with known underlying malignant disease.

Reference

MacMahon H, Austin JH, Gamsu G, et al: Guidelines for management of small pulmonary nodules on CT scans: a statement from the Fleischner Society. *Radiology* 237:395-400, 2005.

Cross-Reference

Thoracic Radiology: THE REQUISITES, 2nd ed, pp 284-286.

Comment

An SPN may represent a benign or malignant lesion. The probability that a nodule is malignant increases according to its size. The likelihood of malignancy in a nodule measuring less than 3 mm is only 0.2%; for nodules measuring 4 to 7 mm, the likelihood increases to 0.9%. Nodules measuring 8 to 20 mm and those measuring greater than 20 mm have a likelihood of malignancy of 18% and 50%, respectively.

More than 50% of all cigarette smokers older than 50 years have at least one pulmonary nodule detected on CT. Cigarette smokers are at greater risk to develop lethal lung cancers than nonsmokers; and their cancer risk increases in proportion to the duration and degree of their smoking. The likelihood of malignancy of an SPN also increases with patient age.

The Fleischner Society published a set of recommendations for the management of incidental solitary pulmonary nodules in 2005 (see Reference). These guidelines apply only to adult patients with nodules that are "incidental," that is, are unrelated to known underlying disease. The guidelines also point out that previous studies (CT scans, chest radiographs) should be obtained, when possible, because they may demonstrate either stability or interval growth of the nodule in question.

Under the Fleischner Society guidelines, the recommended CT follow-up becomes more frequent with increasing nodule size. Furthermore, patients are categorized as "low-risk" (those with a minimal or absent history of smoking and/or other known risk factors) or "high-risk" (those with a history of smoking or of other known risk factors). For individuals in the low-risk category, the recommendations are as follows: nodule 4 mm or less: no follow-up needed; nodule greater than 4 to 6 mm: CT follow-up at 12 months (if unchanged, no further follow-up); nodule greater than 6 to 8 mm: CT at 6 to 12 months, then at 18 to 24 months if no change; nodule greater than 8 mm: CT at 3, 9, and 24 months or PET scan or biopsy.

For individuals in the high-risk category, the recommendations are as follows: nodule 4 mm or less: CT follow-up at 12 months (if unchanged, no further follow-up); nodule greater than 4 to 6 mm: CT follow-up at 6 to 12 months, then 18 to 24 months if no change; nodule greater than 6 to 8 mm: CT at 3 to 6 months, then at 9 to 12 and 24 months if no change; nodule greater than 8 mm: same as for low-risk patient.

The guidelines also point out that nonsolid (ground-glass) or partly solid nodules may require longer follow-up to exclude an indolent adenocarcinoma.

Notes

1. Names at least four causes of tracheal narrowing.

2. Is post-intubation tracheal narrowing typically focal or diffuse?

3. What are some of the presenting symptoms of central airway obstruction?

4. What is the best imaging modality for detection of tracheal stenosis?

CASE 104

Tracheal Stenosis

1. Post-intubation injury, malignant neoplasm, tuberculosis, Wegener's granulomatosis, amyloidosis.

2. Focal.

3. Cough, stridor, wheezing.

4. MDCT with multiplanar and three-dimensional renderings.

Reference

Lee KS, Yoon JH, Kim TK, et al: Evaluation of tracheobronchial disease with helical CT with multiplanar and three dimensional reconstruction: correlation with bronchoscopy. *Radiographics* 17:555-567, 1997.

Cross-Reference

Thoracic Radiology: THE REQUISITES, 2nd ed, pp 290-299.

Comment

Tracheal stricture is the most common late complication of tracheal intubation and decannulation. In the illustrated case, the stenosis manifests as a characteristic focal, short-segment circumferential stenosis at the site of a previous tracheostomy. Tracheal stenosis, tracheomalacia, or an ulcerative tracheoesophageal fistula may develop at the stomal site, at the level of an endotracheal tube cuff, or at the site where the tip of a tracheal tube rests against the tracheal wall. Overdistention of an endotracheal tube cuff may produce pressure necrosis of the tracheal wall. Anterior angulation of an endotracheal tube may produce erosion of the tracheal wall and lead to perforation of the wall and even of the adjacent innominate artery; posterior angulation may result in a tracheoesophageal fistula.

On imaging studies, tracheal stenosis typically manifests as an hourglass-like stenosis. Tracheal stenosis may be missed on conventional chest radiography, and a negative radiograph does not exclude the diagnosis. MDCT is the imaging modality of choice and should include multiplanar and three-dimensional renderings when possible.

Notes

B   In Phase

C   Out of Phase

1. Describe the normal configuration and location of the thymus gland on axial CT imaging.

2. Describe the range of CT attenuation values (Hounsfield units) of the normal thymus on CT imaging.

3. Name at least three causes of thymic hyperplasia.

4. Which imaging modality is most useful for distinguishing thymic hyperplasia from thymic neoplasia?

Thymic Hyperplasia

1. Bilobed, "arrowhead" configuration in the prevascular region of the anterior mediastinum.

2. Soft tissue, soft tissue with fat (speckled), fatty replacement.

3. Myasthenia gravis, rebound thymic hyperplasia following chemotherapy or steroids, hyperthyroidism (Graves' disease), rheumatoid arthritis, scleroderma, red cell aplasia.

4. MRI using a chemical shift technique.

Reference

Inaoka T, Takahashi K, Mineta M, et al: Thymic hyperplasia and thymus gland tumors: differentiation with chemical shift MR imaging. *Radiology* 243:869-876, 2007.

Cross-Reference

Thoracic Radiology: THE REQUISITES, 2nd ed, pp 348-349.

Comment

The normal thymus decreases in size with age as it undergoes fatty infiltration; it is visualized in less than 50% of patients older than 40 years on CT and/or MRI studies. The normal thymus manifests in the prevascular region of the anterior mediastinum as a bilobed homogeneous structure of soft tissue attenuation on CT. With progressive involution and fatty infiltration, it may appear speckled and lobular in configuration.

Thymic enlargement may represent thymic hyperplasia or a thymic epithelial tumor. True thymic hyperplasia represents an increase in size and weight of the thymus with retention of its normal gross architecture and histologic appearance. This form of hyperplasia may occur as a rebound phenomenon following chemotherapy, steroid therapy, or recovery from a severe systemic stress or insult ("rebound thymic hyperplasia"). *Lymphoid (follicular) hyperplasia* refers to a distinct entity characterized by an increased number of lymphoid follicles that is not usually associated with thymic enlargement. It is most commonly associated with myasthenia gravis, but is also associated with autoimmune and systemic disorders, including hyperthyroidism (Graves' disease), acromegaly, systemic lupus erythematosus, scleroderma, rheumatoid arthritis, and cirrhosis.

Chemical-shift MRI is a recently developed technique that may be helpful in distinguishing thymic hyperplasia from thymoma and other thymic epithelial tumors. In this technique, comparison between in-phase and out-of-phase gradient-echo images reveals homogeneously decreased signal intensity in normal thymus and thymic hyperplasia on out-of-phase images due to diffuse fatty infiltration, as shown in this case. In contrast, thymic epithelial neoplasms usually do not exhibit this pattern.

Notes

1. Regarding solitary pulmonary nodules (SPNs), which is most likely to be malignant: a solid nodule, a ground-glass nodule, or a semi-solid nodule of mixed attenuation (ground-glass and solid components)?

2. What focal disease entities manifest most commonly on imaging studies as a solid nodule with a halo of surrounding ground-glass opacity?

3. In which clinical setting is invasive aspergillosis most likely to occur?

4. Bronchioloalveolar carcinoma (BAC) is a subtype of which lung cancer cell type?

Mixed Attenuation SPN

1. A semi-solid nodule of mixed attenuation.

2. BAC, invasive aspergillosis, candidiasis, cytomegalovirus.

3. Severely neutropenic patient.

4. Adenocarcinoma.

Reference

Müller NL, Silva CIS: Nodules and masses. In: Silva CIS, Müller NL, Eds. *Imaging of the Chest*. Philadelphia: Saunders, 2008, pp 136-157.

Cross-Reference

Thoracic Radiology: THE REQUISITES, 2nd ed, pp 284-286.

Comment

On thin-section CT, a malignant SPN may be of soft tissue or ground-glass attenuation, or a combination of both ground-glass and solid components (i.e., semi-solid or mixed attenuation). Of those patterns, the mixed attenuation (semi-solid) solitary nodule is the most likely to be malignant, and the soft tissue nodule is the most likely to be benign.

A mixed attenuation nodule with a halo of surrounding ground-glass opacity is also an imaging manifestations of invasive aspergillosis and candidiasis, typically occurring in a severely neutropenic patient, and of cytomegalovirus, most commonly occurring 1 month or longer following organ transplantation.

Besides the variability of their CT attenuation, malignant SPNs are also variable in their border characteristics and may manifest as spiculated, ill-defined, or well-defined nodular opacities.

Notes

Challenge

1. Name at least three entities that typically present with a peripheral distribution of consolidation.

2. Which entity is most closely associated with a "photographic negative of pulmonary edema" pattern?

3. How is this disorder treated?

4. What percentage of patients with chronic eosinophilic pneumonia have a history of asthma?

Chronic Eosinophilic Pneumonia

1. Löffler's syndrome, chronic eosinophilic pneumonia, cryptogenic organizing pneumonia (COP), pulmonary infarcts, vasculitides.

2. Chronic eosinophilic pneumonia.

3. Steroids.

4. About 50%.

Reference

Jeong YJ, Kim K, Seo IJ, et al: Eosinophilic lung diseases: a clinical, radiologic, and pathologic overview. *Radiographics* 27:617-637, 2007.

Cross-Reference

Thoracic Radiology: THE REQUISITES, 2nd ed, pp 228-229.

Comment

The chest radiograph in this case demonstrates multifocal areas of consolidation in both lungs, with a striking peripheral predominance in the upper lobes (best demonstrated on the coned-down image in the second figure). The distribution is typical of chronic eosinophilic pneumonia.

Affected patients typically present with symptoms of dyspnea, fever, chills, night sweats, and weight loss. Symptoms are usually present for an average of nearly 8 months prior to diagnosis. Women are affected more frequently than men, and there is a history of asthma in about one half of cases. Eosinophilia is present in the majority of patients and is usually mild to moderate.

The typical radiographic appearance is a peripheral pattern of consolidation, often with an apical or axillary distribution. The lung bases are less frequently involved. Also note the presence of right basilar consolidation in the first figure. In some patients, the opacities resolve and recur in the same location. When peripheral consolidation surrounds the lungs, the pattern is referred to as a *photographic negative of pulmonary edema*. Pleural effusions (which are present in this case) are infrequently encountered (less than 10% of cases).

Affected patients usually show a rapid response to steroid therapy, with clinical improvement within hours and radiographic resolution within days.

Notes

1. Name the structure that communicates with this cyst.

2. Is this a common location for this entity?

3. How can you differentiate this structure from an apical lung hernia?

4. Is this location typical for this entity?

Right Paratracheal Air Cyst (Diverticulum)

1. Trachea.

2. Yes.

3. Only an apical lung hernia is contiguous with the lung and demonstrates lung architectural features.

4. Yes.

Reference

Buterbaugh JE, Erly WK: Paratracheal air cysts: a common finding on routine CT examinations of the cervical spine and neck that may mimic pneumomediastinum in patients with traumatic injuries. *AJNR Am J Neuroradiol* 29:1218-1221, 2008.

Cross-Reference

None.

Comment

The conventional tomogram in the first figure demonstrates a well-marginated, septated cystic structure in the right paratracheal region adjacent to the right lung apex. The differential diagnosis includes a right paratracheal air cyst, apical bullae, and an apical lung hernia. The CT image in the second figure demonstrates that the cystic structure is mediastinal in location, directly communicates with the right posterolateral wall of the trachea, and does not demonstrate lung architectural features. The imaging characteristics are typical of a large right paratracheal air cyst, an abnormality of the trachea that is thought to represent a tracheal diverticulum.

Such diverticula occur most commonly at the right posterolateral wall of the trachea at the level of the thoracic inlet and vary in size from a few millimeters to several centimeters. Although once considered relatively rare, small diverticula are recognized with increased frequency with modern multidetector CT (MDCT) scanners and have been reported in about 4% of neck CT scans of children and adults that included the thoracic inlet region. In the setting of trauma, a small diverticulum may potentially mimic pneumomediastinum, but its characteristic location and appearance should allow for an accurate diagnosis.

It has been proposed that acquired tracheal diverticula may occur in response to raised intratracheal pressures related to repeated bouts of coughing in patients with chronic respiratory disorders such as emphysema. However, many diverticula are considered to be congenital in etiology and are incidentally detected in both children and adults. Although usually asymptomatic, patients with diverticula may rarely present with clinical symptoms of prolonged productive cough, hemoptysis, and chest pain. Symptomatic lesions are treated surgically, but asymptomatic diverticula require no intervention.

Notes

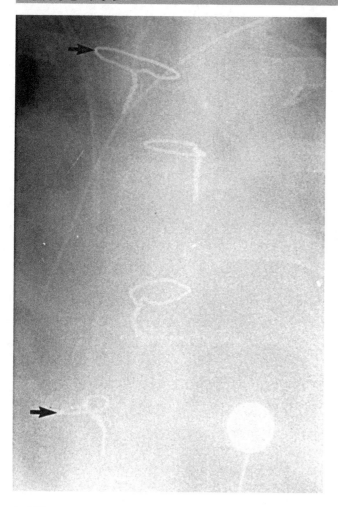

1. What postoperative complication is present in this case?

2. Is this a serious complication?

3. How is this complication treated?

4. What sternal wire abnormality is most commonly seen on postoperative radiographs in patients with this complication?

Sternal Dehiscence Following Median Sternotomy

1. Sternal dehiscence.

2. Yes.

3. Reoperation for sternal closure.

4. Sternal wire displacement.

Reference

Boiselle PM, Mansilla AV, Fisher MS, McLoud TC: Wandering wires: frequency of sternal wire abnormalities in patients with sternal dehiscence. *AJR Am J Roentgenol* 173:777-780, 1999.

Cross-Reference

None.

Comment

Following median sternotomy, the sternal wires are typically maintained in a vertical row along the midline of the sternum. The coned-down chest radiograph shows a scrambled arrangement of the sternal wires, with the first and fourth wires displaced to the right of the midline *(arrows)*. Displacement of sternal wires is a highly sensitive and specific sign for sternal dehiscence, an uncommon but serious complication following median sternotomy.

Although sternal dehiscence is often evident on the basis of physical examination findings, it may be clinically occult in some cases. Sternal wire abnormalities, most notably displacement, are seen in the majority of patients with this condition; importantly, such abnormalities may precede the clinical diagnosis in some cases. Thus, when reviewing postoperative radiographs of a patient who is status post median sternotomy, you should carefully assess the sternal wires. Interval displacement or rotation of one or more wires (in comparison with their appearance on the first postoperative radiograph) should prompt careful clinical assessment for signs of dehiscence.

The high frequency of sternal wire displacement in patients with sternal dehiscence fits well with the proposed mechanism of this complication. It has been proposed that sternal separation is the result of sternal sutures pulling or cutting through the sternum rather than breaking. As the sternum separates, some sutures will travel with the right side of the sternum and others will migrate to the left side. The term *wandering wires* has been used to describe the characteristic alterations in sternal wires on radiographs of patients with sternal dehiscence.

Notes

1. What is the most likely cause for the mediastinal fluid collection in this septic patient who is 18 days status post median sternotomy?

2. In the postoperative setting, are the CT findings of localized retrosternal fluid collections and pneumomediastinum highly sensitive for mediastinitis?

3. Are these findings highly specific in the early postoperative period?

4. At what time point after surgery does the specificity of this finding increase?

C A S E   1 1 0

Postoperative Mediastinitis

1. Mediastinitis.

2. Yes.

3. No.

4. After 14 days.

Reference

Jolles H, Henry DA, Robertson JF, et al: Mediastinitis following median sternotomy: CT findings. *Radiology* 201:463-466, 1996.

Cross-Reference

Thoracic Radiology: THE REQUISITES, 2nd ed, pp 370-371.

Comment

Mediastinitis is a relatively uncommon but serious complication following median sternotomy. *Mediastinitis* refers to inflammation and infection of the mediastinum and is a more serious complication than superficial infection localized to the peristernal soft tissue structures of the chest wall.

The CT diagnosis of mediastinitis is based primarily on the presence of mediastinal air and fluid collections. It is important to be aware that such findings can be seen normally in the early postoperative period in patients without mediastinitis.

In a study of patients with postoperative mediastinitis by Jolles and colleagues, it was reported that the CT findings of localized mediastinal fluid and pneumomediastinum *(arrow)* are highly sensitive (100%) for mediastinitis. The specificity of these findings is quite low (33%) within the first 14 days following surgery but increases significantly (100%) after postoperative day 14. Thus, when evaluating the CT scan of a postoperative patient with suspected mediastinitis, you must correlate CT findings with the time interval since surgery.

Although these data suggest that CT is most helpful in the late postoperative period, there is a role for CT imaging in the early postoperative period as well. For example, a negative CT scan of the mediastinum can be useful for directing attention to other sites of possible infection. Moreover, the identification of localized retrosternal fluid collections may be helpful for guiding aspiration procedures in patients in whom there is a strong clinical suspicion for mediastinitis.

Notes

A

B

1. What is the most likely cause for these serial radiographic findings that developed within 1 week following right upper lobe resection for lung cancer?

2. What type of organism is most commonly responsible for nosocomial pneumonia?

3. What term is used to describe cavitary pneumonia associated with intracavitary sloughed lung?

4. What organism is most closely associated with this entity?

Pulmonary Gangrene Secondary to
Klebsiella Pneumonia

1. Pneumonia.

2. Gram-negative organisms.

3. Pulmonary gangrene.

4. *Klebsiella*.

Reference
Tzeng DZ, Markman M, Hardin K: Necrotizing pneumonia and pulmonary gangrene: difficulty in diagnosis, evaluation and treatment. *Clin Pulm Med* 14:166-170, 2007.

Cross-Reference
Thoracic Radiology: THE REQUISITES, 2nd ed, p 84.

Comment
Nosocomial pneumonia is most commonly caused by gram-negative organisms. Hospitalized patients at increased risk for nosocomial pneumonia include patients who are maintained on artificial ventilators and those who have intravenous catheters and other forms of ancillary support devices.

Pneumonia may be complicated by lung necrosis and cavitation, particularly when it is caused by virulent organisms. Bacteria that frequently cause cavitation include *Staphylococcus aureus*, gram-negative bacteria, anaerobic bacteria, and *Mycobacterium tuberculosis*. When necrosis is extensive, arteritis and vascular thrombosis may develop in an area of intense inflammation, resulting in ischemic necrosis and death of a portion of the lung. This process may result in the presence of sloughed lung within a cavity (second figure) and is referred to as *pulmonary gangrene*. You should not confuse this entity with the "ball-in-cavity" appearance that is associated with the saprophytic form of *Aspergillus* infection. An aspergilloma develops within a long-standing, preexisting cavity. In contrast, in pulmonary gangrene, a cavity and intracavitary sloughed lung develop rapidly within an area of acute consolidation.

Although pulmonary gangrene is most closely associated with *Klebsiella*, it is not specific for this organism. This entity has been described in association with a variety of other organisms, including *Streptococcus pneumoniae*, *M. tuberculosis*, and *Mucormycetes*, among others.

Notes

1. What is the distribution of emphysema in this patient?

2. Is this distribution typical of emphysema related to cigarette smoking?

3. Name the four basic types of emphysema.

4. Name at least one cause of panlobular emphysema with a basilar predominance.

Panlobular Emphysema Secondary to Intravenous Methylphenidate

1. Lower lobe predominance.

2. No.

3. Centrilobular, panlobular, paraseptal, and paracicatricial.

4. Alpha$_1$-antitrypsin (AAT) deficiency and intravenous injection of methylphenidate (Ritalin).

Reference

Hagan IG, Burney K: Radiology of recreational drug abuse. *Radiographics* 27:919-940, 2007.

Cross-Reference

Thoracic Radiology: THE REQUISITES, 2nd ed, pp 242-248.

Comment

Emphysema is defined by the presence of abnormal, permanent enlargement of the airspaces distal to the terminal bronchiole, accompanied by destruction of their walls without obvious fibrosis.

The radiograph demonstrates hyperinflation of the lungs with associated reduced vascularity in the lower lobes. The high-resolution CT (HRCT) image reveals extensive areas of abnormal low attenuation in the lower lobes with a paucity of pulmonary vessels. The CT appearance is typical of *panlobular emphysema,* which has been described as a "diffuse simplification of lung architecture." Panlobular emphysema is almost always most severe in the lower lobes. In contrast, *centrilobular emphysema* is usually most prominent in the upper lobes.

AAT deficiency is the most common cause of panlobular emphysema with a lower lobe predominance. Intravenous drug abusers who inject methylphenidate may develop a basilar distribution of panlobular emphysema that is indistinguishable radiographically from AAT deficiency. The pathogenesis of emphysema in such patients is unknown. This condition can be distinguished from AAT deficiency by a history of methylphenidate injection, normal AAT serum levels, and pathologic evidence of microscopic talc granulomas.

Interestingly, large upper lobe bullae have been reported in individuals who regularly smoke marijuana. The mechanism is thought to involve a combination of direct pulmonary toxicity along with pleural pressure changes and airway barotrauma related to high inspiratory pressures associated with smoking marijuana.

Notes

A   Inspiration

B   Expiration

1. In a patient who is status post bone marrow transplantation, what is the most likely cause for these inspiratory and expiratory HRCT findings?

2. Name three CT findings that may be associated with obliterative bronchiolitis (OB).

3. Is OB a constrictive or a proliferative form of bronchiolitis?

4. Name at least four diseases or conditions that may be associated with OB.

Obliterative Bronchiolitis

1. OB.

2. Mosaic perfusion, bronchial dilation, and air trapping.

3. Constrictive.

4. Bone marrow transplantation, viral infections, toxic fume inhalation, rheumatoid arthritis, lung transplantation, and inflammatory bowel disease.

Reference

Silva CI, Müller NL: Obliterative bronchiolitis. In: Boiselle PM, Lynch DA, Eds. *CT of the Airways.* Totowa NJ, Humana, 2008, pp 293-323.

Cross-Reference

Thoracic Radiology: THE REQUISITES, 2nd ed, pp 321-325.

Comment

The inspiratory HRCT image in the first figure reveals a subtle pattern of variable lung attenuation, with a slight decrease in the caliber and number of pulmonary vessels within the areas of low attenuation. This appearance has been referred to as a *mosaic pattern* of lung attenuation and may be encountered in patients with small airways disease and pulmonary vascular abnormalities such as chronic pulmonary embolism. The expiratory HRCT image in the second figure demonstrates extensive air trapping, a finding that distinguishes small airways disease from pulmonary vascular disease.

A mosaic pattern of lung attenuation with air trapping on expiratory scans is the hallmark of OB. OB is characterized histologically by concentric narrowing of the bronchioles by submucosal and peribronchiolar fibrosis. Affected patients typically present with dyspnea. Pulmonary function tests reveal a progressive, nonreversible airflow obstruction pattern.

A variety of conditions are associated with OB, including bone marrow transplantation. Approximately 10% of bone marrow transplant patients develop OB. In such patients, this condition is thought to be related to chronic graft-versus-host disease and has a high mortality rate.

Other conditions associated with OB include childhood respiratory infections, chronic rejection following lung and heart-lung transplantation, post inhalational, ingested toxins, connective tissue disorders, drugs, inflammatory bowel disease, and a variety of miscellaneous conditions.

Notes

A

B

1. Name the condition that is characterized by multiple pulmonary nodules and masses in a patient who is status post prior hysterectomy for uterine fibroids.

2. What is the typical time course for pulmonary lesions associated with this condition?

3. Name at least one other neoplasm that is characterized by extremely slowly growing pulmonary metastases.

4. Name at least two neoplasms that are associated with rapidly growing pulmonary metastases.

Metastasizing Leiomyoma

1. Metastasizing leiomyoma.

2. Slow.

3. Thyroid carcinoma, salivary gland neoplasms.

4. Sarcomas, melanomas, and germ cell neoplasms.

Reference

Abrahamson S, Gilkeson RC, Goldstein JD, et al: Benign metastasizing leiomyoma: clinical, imaging, and pathologic correlation. *AJR Am J Roentgenol* 176:1409-1413, 2001.

Cross-Reference

Thoracic Radiology: THE REQUISITES, 2nd ed, pp 278-282.

Comment

Pulmonary metastases are an important cause of multiple lung nodules and masses. Such nodules and masses are usually peripheral in location and have a basilar predominance.

Leiomyomas are an uncommon cause of pulmonary metastases. Other less common potential sites of involvement include lymph nodes, peritoneum, and retroperitoneal structures. The behavior of such lesions varies from that of a benign lesion to a low-grade sarcoma. Thus, the more general term *metastasizing leiomyoma* is preferable to the phrase "benign metastasizing leiomyoma."

In women, these lesions may be very slowly growing metastases from a uterine leiomyoma. Affected patients often have a history of previous hysterectomy for uterine fibroids. The pulmonary lesions are usually very sensitive to hormonal therapy.

Notes

A

B

1. What is the term used to describe the curvilinear opacity in the first figure that courses parallel to the pleural surface?

2. What is the term used to describe the long linear opacities in the second figure that course perpendicular to the pleural surface?

3. With what chronic infiltrative lung disease are these findings most closely associated?

4. Are they pathognomonic for this process?

Asbestosis

1. Subpleural curvilinear line.

2. Parenchymal bands.

3. Asbestosis.

4. No.

Reference

Staples CA: Computed tomography in the evaluation of benign asbestos-related disorders. *Radiol Clin North Am* 30:1191-1207, 1992.

Cross-Reference

Thoracic Radiology: THE REQUISITES, 2nd ed, pp 209-213.

Comment

Asbestosis refers to pulmonary fibrosis that occurs in asbestos workers. It usually occurs in individuals who have been exposed to high concentrations over a prolonged period. Affected patients typically present with symptoms of a dry cough and dyspnea. Pulmonary function tests reveal a progressive reduction in vital capacity and diffusing capacity.

On conventional radiographs, you may observe a linear or reticular pattern of parenchymal opacities in the lower lung zones, which may progress to honeycombing. The identification of pleural plaques or pleural thickening supports the diagnosis (note pleural thickening in the figures). However, pleural abnormalities may be absent. It is important to recognize that normal conventional radiographs do not exclude a diagnosis of asbestosis.

CT, particularly HRCT, is superior to radiography in the detection, quantification, and characterization of asbestosis. HRCT findings include (1) subpleural curvilinear lines; (2) thickened septal lines (the most common finding); (3) subpleural dependent density; (4) parenchymal bands; and (5) honeycombing. In an asbestos-exposed individual with a normal chest radiograph, these HRCT findings are suggestive of asbestosis; however, they are not specific for this process.

Notes

A

B

1. In this patient with a history of prior right pneumonectomy, how can you explain the presence of aerated lung in the right hemithorax?

2. Why do you think that this patient is experiencing dyspnea?

3. Is the post-pneumonectomy syndrome more common following right or left pneumonectomy?

4. How is this syndrome treated?

Post-pneumonectomy Syndrome

1. Herniation of the left upper lobe into the right hemithorax.

2. Compression of the left lower lobe bronchus by vascular structures.

3. Right.

4. Surgical repositioning of the mediastinal structures and placement of a saline prosthesis in the pneumonectomy space.

Reference

Shen KR, Wain JC, Wright DC, et al: Postpneumonectomy syndrome: surgical management and long-term results. *J Thorac Cardiovasc Surg* 135:1210-1216, 2008.

Cross-Reference

None.

Comment

Post-pneumonectomy syndrome is a rare, delayed complication following pneumonectomy, often performed at an early age. It is more common following right pneumonectomy than left pneumonectomy. Affected patients present with symptoms of dyspnea and recurrent infections in the remaining lung.

The syndrome occurs secondary to marked mediastinal shift, rotation of the heart and great vessels, and herniation of the remaining lung into the contralateral side of the chest. Following realignment of these structures, the airway may be compressed (*arrow,* second figure) by the thoracic spine, descending thoracic aorta, ligamentum arteriosum, and pulmonary artery.

CT plays an important role in delineating the presence and cause of airway obstruction. Inspiratory-expiratory CT may also assess for the presence of tracheobronchomalacia, an important preoperative finding. Prompt diagnosis and treatment are important, because surgical results are favorable before malacic changes have occurred within the obstructed airway.

Notes

1. What is Mounier-Kuhn syndrome?

2. What is the radiologic definition of tracheomegaly?

3. What does the *curved arrow* in the second figure represent?

4. Is this a common location for this finding?

C A S E 1 1 7

Mounier-Kuhn Syndrome With Tracheal Diverticulum

1. An entity characterized by congenital tracheobronchomegaly and recurrent respiratory infections.

2. A coronal tracheal diameter of greater than 25 mm in men and greater than 21 mm in women, as measured 2 cm above the aortic arch on a standard posteroanterior (PA) erect chest radiograph.

3. A tracheal diverticulum.

4. Yes.

Reference
Boiselle PM: Tracheal abnormalities: tracheomegaly. In: Müller NL, Silva CI, Eds. *Imaging of the Chest*. Philadelphia, Saunders, 2008, pp 1014-1017.

Cross-Reference
Thoracic Radiology: THE REQUISITES, 2nd ed, pp 59, 61, 299-300.

Comment
Mounier-Kuhn syndrome, also referred to as *congenital tracheobronchomegaly,* is characterized pathologically by atrophy or absence of elastic fibers and thinning of the muscular mucosa of the trachea and main bronchi. This results in a flaccid airway that abnormally dilates during inspiration and excessively collapses on expiration. An ineffective coughing mechanism and pooling of secretions within outpouchings of mucosa predispose affected patients to recurrent bouts of respiratory infections. Pulmonary complications include bronchiectasis, emphysema, and pulmonary fibrosis. Note the presence of tracheomegaly (note 4.2-cm-diameter coronal dimension), cystic bronchiectasis, and emphysema in the first figure.

The second figure reveals an enlarged trachea and a wide-mouthed tracheal diverticulum *(curved arrow).* The posterolateral wall of the trachea is the most common location for a diverticulum in patients with Mounier-Kuhn syndrome. This site represents the junction of the posterior membranous and the anterior cartilaginous portions of the trachea. A minority of patients with Mounier-Kuhn syndrome demonstrate widespread tracheal and bronchial diverticula.

Other associations with primary tracheomegaly include Ehlers-Danlos syndrome, Marfan syndrome, and cutis laxa. Secondary tracheomegaly may develop in patients with long-standing pulmonary fibrosis, possibly secondary to chronic coughing and recurrent infections.

Notes

1. What is the most common cause of central bronchiectasis?

2. What other imaging findings are associated with allergic bronchopulmonary aspergillosis (ABPA)?

3. What types of patients are predisposed to this condition?

4. Characterize the type of bronchiectasis in this case (cylindrical, varicose, or cystic).

CASE 118

Allergic Bronchopulmonary Aspergillosis

1. ABPA.

2. Mucoid impaction, recurrent atelectasis, patchy consolidation.

3. Asthmatics.

4. Varicose.

Reference

Franquet T, Müller NL, Oikonomou A, Flint JD: *Aspergillus* infection of the airways: computed tomography and pathologic findings. *J Comput Assist Tomogr* 28:10-16, 2004.

Cross-Reference

Thoracic Radiology: THE REQUISITES, 2nd ed, pp 114, 250, 251, 314, 321, 322.

Comment

ABPA is a hypersensitivity reaction that occurs when *Aspergillus* organisms are inhaled by an atopic individual. The inhaled fungus grows in a noninvasive manner within the bronchi and incites an allergic response. The bronchi become dilated and filled with mucus that contains abundant eosinophils and fragmented fungal hyphae.

Affected patients typically have a history of asthma. Presenting signs and symptoms may include fever, pleuritic chest pain, expectoration of mucous plugs, and chronic cough. Radiographic features include central bronchiectasis, mucous plugging ("finger-in-glove" appearance), atelectasis, and patchy, migratory foci of consolidation.

The most characteristic imaging finding is mucous plugging. As the mucous plugs are expectorated, dilated, air-filled bronchi can be identified, especially on CT scans. The central bronchi are most commonly affected and typically demonstrate a varicoid appearance.

Because ABPA is an allergic disease, treatment consists of steroids. Chronic cases may be complicated by upper lobe scarring and bronchiectasis.

Notes

1. What HRCT findings are associated with the term *crazy-paving*?

2. Name the disorder that is classically associated with this pattern.

3. Name three pulmonary infections that may complicate pulmonary alveolar proteinosis (PAP).

4. How is PAP treated?

Pulmonary Alveolar Proteinosis

1. Ground-glass opacity with superimposed smooth septal thickening in a patchy or geographic distribution.

2. PAP.

3. Infection with *Nocardia*, *Aspergillus*, and *Mucormycetes*.

4. Bronchoalveolar lavage (BAL).

Reference
Rossi SE, Erasmus JJ, Volpacchio M, et al: "Crazy-paving" pattern at thin-section CT of the lungs: radiologic-pathologic overview. *Radiographics* 23:1509-1519, 2003.

Cross-Reference
Thoracic Radiology: THE REQUISITES, 2nd ed, pp 198-199.

Comment
PAP is characterized by filling of the alveolar spaces with periodic acid–Schiff (PAS)–positive proteinaceous material, with little or no associated tissue reaction. The cause of PAP is unknown, but is has been suggested that the underlying mechanism is excessive production or impaired removal of surfactant. Although most cases are idiopathic, PAP has been reported to occur in association with an overwhelming exposure to silica and in association with immunologic disturbances.

PAP typically affects men in the fourth and fifth decades of life, and presenting symptoms include a non-productive cough and dyspnea. Chest radiographic findings are often striking and consist of alveolar consolidation and ground-glass opacification in a symmetric, bilateral, perihilar distribution. On HRCT, ground-glass opacification predominates, and it is often patchy or geographic. A "crazy-paving" pattern is formed when smoothly thickened interlobular septal lines are superimposed on ground-glass opacification.

The prognosis of PAP has improved since the advent of therapy with BAL, which is successful in most cases. However, some patients require retreatment for relapse, and a minority of patients eventually become refractory to treatment.

Notes

1. Define tracheomalacia.

2. What do patients with primary (congenital) tracheomalacia lack?

3. During which phase of respiration is tracheal collapsibility most apparent?

4. What term is used to describe the inspiratory tracheal shape demonstrated in the first figure?

Tracheomalacia

1. Excessive collapsibility of the trachea secondary to weakness of the tracheal walls and supporting cartilages.

2. Cartilage.

3. Expiration.

4. Lunate trachea (defined as coronal diameter greater than sagittal diameter).

Reference

Lee EY, Litmanovich D, Boiselle PM: Multidetector CT evaluation of tracheobronchomalacia. *Radiol Clin North Am* 47:261-269, 2009.

Cross-Reference

Thoracic Radiology: THE REQUISITES, 2nd ed, pp 59, 61, 302-304.

Comment

Tracheobronchomalacia refers to excessive collapsibility of the airway. Such collapsibility is usually most apparent during coughing and during forced expiration. The abnormally flaccid airway is associated with physiologic alterations, including an inefficient coughing mechanism and retained secretions. This may lead to recurrent infections and bronchiectasis. Rarely, it may be complicated by respiratory failure.

A primary cause of tracheobronchomalacia is congenital deficiency of cartilage. Acquired causes include prior intubation, chronic obstructive pulmonary disease (COPD), trauma, infection, relapsing polychondritis, and extrinsic compression (e.g., from a thyroid goiter).

Patients with severely symptomatic tracheomalacia may potentially benefit from surgery such as tracheoplasty, a technique that involves reinforcement of the posterior membranous wall of the trachea with a graft. This procedure has shown promising results in patients with acquired tracheomalacia in whom excessive tracheal collapsibility is mostly due to an abnormally flaccid posterior tracheal wall.

Notes

1. What are the two most common cell types of primary malignant tracheal neoplasms?

2. Which of the two cell types is more common in cigarette smokers?

3. Which of the two cell types has a better prognosis?

4. In general, what degree of tracheal luminal narrowing must be present before patients are symptomatic from a primary tracheal malignancy?

Adenoid Cystic Carcinoma of the Trachea

1. Squamous cell carcinoma and adenoid cystic carcinoma.

2. Squamous cell carcinoma.

3. Adenoid cystic carcinoma.

4. A reduction to approximately 25% of the normal tracheal luminal area.

Reference

Lee KS, Boiselle PM: Tracheal and bronchial neoplasms. In: Boiselle PM, Lynch D, Eds. *CT of the Airways.* Totowa NJ, Humana, 2008, pp 151-190.

Cross-Reference

Thoracic Radiology: THE REQUISITES, 2nd ed, pp 301-303.

Comment

Primary tracheal neoplasms are quite rare. In adult patients, the majority of tracheal neoplasms are malignant. Presenting symptoms include shortness of breath and wheezing. Affected patients may be initially misdiagnosed with adult-onset asthma. This diagnosis should prompt you to carefully assess the airway on chest radiographs!

Squamous cell carcinoma has a male predilection, and it is strongly associated with cigarette smoking. Squamous cell carcinoma is associated with a poor prognosis. Therapy consists of surgery and radiation for localized disease and radiation alone for surgically unresectable cases.

Adenoid cystic carcinoma is a low-grade malignancy that has no gender predilection and no relationship to cigarette smoking. Adenoid cystic carcinoma has a significantly better prognosis than squamous cell carcinoma, and surgical resection is potentially curative for patients with localized disease. Adjuvant radiation therapy is often required because of the predilection for these tumors to spread perineurally and submucosally. Late recurrences and metastases have been reported, however, especially among patients treated only with radiation therapy.

MDCT plays an important role in preoperative planning of tracheal neoplasms by determining the amenability of a lesion to complete resection and by guiding the surgeon with respect to the approach, type, and extent of resection. Multiplanar reformation and three-dimensional reconstruction images play a complementary role to axial images by enhancing the accurate assessment of the craniocaudal extent of a neoplasm and its relationship to adjacent mediastinal structures.

Notes

A

B

1. What are the two most common causes of a tubular opacity in the lung?

2. List two entities that are commonly associated with mucoid impaction.

3. What is the most common cell type of non–small cell lung cancer to present as an endobronchial lesion?

4. When mucoid impaction occurs secondary to bronchial obstruction, how does the adjacent lung remain aerated?

Mucoid Impaction Secondary to Bronchial Obstruction (Squamous Cell Carcinoma)

1. Mucoid impaction and arteriovenous malformation.

2. Allergic bronchopulmonary aspergillosis (ABPA) and cystic fibrosis.

3. Squamous cell carcinoma.

4. Collateral air drift.

Reference
Martinez S, Heyneman LE, McAdams HP, et al: Mucoid impactions: finger-in-glove sign and other CT and radiographic features. *Radiographics* 28:1369-1382, 2008.

Cross-Reference
Thoracic Radiology: THE REQUISITES, 2nd ed, p 318.

Comment
Mucoid impaction manifests on imaging studies as tubular or branching tubular Y- and V-shaped opacities, sometimes described as resembling a "finger-in-glove" appearance. Mucoid impaction is most often associated with ABPA and cystic fibrosis. It is important to be aware that mucoid impaction can also occur distal to a bronchial obstruction from both malignant (e.g., lung cancer, bronchial carcinoid) and benign (e.g., tuberculosis [TB] bronchostenosis) etiologies. In such cases, the affected portion of the lung remains aerated secondary to collateral air drift through interalveolar connections (pores of Kohn) and bronchiole-alveolar connections (canals of Lambert).

Detection of a tubular opacity on chest radiography should prompt consideration of both mucoid impaction and arteriovenous malformation as potential diagnoses. They can usually be distinguished on CT scans by assessing the bronchi, that is, in cases of arteriovenous malformation a normal bronchus may be observed adjacent to the tubular opacity. In some cases, low CT density numbers (−5 to +20) can confirm the diagnosis of mucoid impaction. If the diagnosis remains in doubt, contrast-enhanced CT can readily differentiate between these entities, because only an arteriovenous malformation enhances with contrast.

Notes

1. Are all localized fibrous tumors of the pleura histologically benign?

2. Are localized fibrous tumors of the pleura related to asbestos exposure?

3. Name a skeletal abnormality that is associated with localized fibrous tumors of the pleura.

4. What is the typical signal intensity of fibrous tumors of the pleura on T1W and T2W MRI?

Localized Fibrous Tumor of the Pleura

1. No.

2. No.

3. Hypertrophic osteoarthropathy.

4. Low signal intensity on T1W and T2W.

Reference

Rosado-de-Christenson ML, Abbott GF, McAdams HP, et al: From the archives of the AFIP: localized fibrous tumor of the pleura. *Radiographics* 23:759-783, 2003.

Cross-Reference

Thoracic Radiology: THE REQUISITES, 2nd ed, pp 389-390, 391.

Comment

Localized fibrous tumors of the pleura (synonym: *solitary fibrous tumors*) are uncommon primary pleural neoplasms. Histologically, approximately 60% are benign and 40% are malignant. However, all lesions are associated with a good prognosis, and the majority are curable by surgical resection.

Affected patients typically present in the sixth to seventh decades of life. In approximately 50% of cases, the patients are asymptomatic. Large lesions may produce symptoms such as cough, dyspnea, and chest pain. In a small minority of cases, patients may present with extra-pulmonary manifestations, including hypertrophic osteo-arthropathy and episodic hypoglycemia.

On chest radiographs, localized fibrous tumors of the pleura typically appear as round or lobulated masses that may have incomplete borders. Such masses vary in size and typically demonstrate a slow growth rate. Lesions attached to the visceral pleura by a pedicle may demonstrate mobility in response to changes in respiration and alterations in patient positioning.

On CT, small fibrous tumors of the pleura are typically homogeneous in attenuation, whereas larger tumors are often heterogeneous, particularly when imaged with contrast enhancement. On MRI, these lesions typically demonstrate low signal intensity on all sequences, reflecting the fibrous content within the stroma of the tumor, but larger tumors may manifest with increased signal on T2W images.

Notes

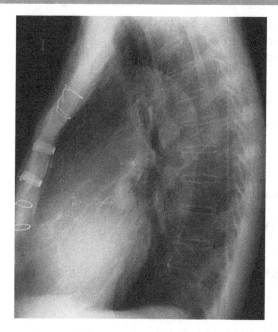

1. In a patient who is status post heart transplantation, is a pulmonary nodule or mass more likely to be neoplastic or infectious in etiology?

2. Infections with which two organisms comprise the majority of lung nodules or masses in heart transplant patients?

3. Name the most common noninfectious etiology of lung nodules or masses in heart transplant patients.

4. Approximately what percentage of heart transplant patients develop posttransplant lymphoproliferative disorder?

Solitary Pulmonary Nodule Secondary to *Nocardia* Infection in a Heart Transplant Patient

1. Infectious.

2. *Aspergillus* and *Nocardia*.

3. Posttransplant lymphoproliferative disorder.

4. Between 2% and 6%.

Reference
Haramati LB, Schulman LL, Austin JHM: Lung nodules and masses after cardiac transplantation. *Radiology* 188:491-497, 1993.

Cross-Reference
Thoracic Radiology: THE REQUISITES, 2nd ed, pp 122-125.

Comment
Cardiac transplantation is currently a widely accepted treatment for end-stage heart disease. The most common causes of morbidity and mortality following heart transplantation are infection and rejection.

When you detect single or multiple lung nodules or masses in a patient who is status post heart transplantation, you should first consider infectious etiologies such as *Aspergillus* and *Nocardia*. In a series of 257 patients who underwent heart transplantation, single or multiple lung nodules or masses were detected on chest radiographs in approximately 10% of patients. Infections were the most common etiology, with *Aspergillus* encountered slightly more frequently than *Nocardia*. *Aspergillus* infection developed a median of 2 months following transplantation, whereas *Nocardia* infection developed a median of 5 months after transplantation.

The time course for susceptibility to specific organisms is similar among patients following heart and other solid organ transplants. In the first month after transplantation, bacterial nosocomial infections are most common. Between 2 and 6 months, viral and opportunistic fungal infections are most common. Once a patient is beyond 6 months posttransplantation, bacterial community-acquired pneumonias are most common.

Posttransplant lymphoproliferative disorder is an important noninfectious cause of lung nodules and masses that is closely associated with the Epstein-Barr virus. The incidence of this disorder is highest during the first year following transplantation, corresponding to the time of most severe immunosuppression. Lung parenchymal abnormalities are frequently accompanied by mediastinal and/or hilar lymph node enlargement, a finding that is not typically associated with *Aspergillus* and *Nocardia* infections.

Notes

1. What is the most likely cause of pulmonary artery hypertension in this patient?

2. Name the term that is used to describe areas of variable lung attenuation with a lobular or multilobular distribution, as shown in the second figure?

3. Is mural thrombus a characteristic feature of acute or chronic pulmonary thromboembolism?

4. Is calcified thrombus a characteristic feature of acute or chronic pulmonary thromboembolism?

Chronic Pulmonary Thromboembolism

1. Chronic pulmonary thromboembolism.

2. Mosaic attenuation pattern.

3. Chronic.

4. Chronic.

Reference

Wittram C, Maher MM, Yoo AJ, et al: CT angiography of pulmonary embolism: diagnostic criteria and causes of misdiagnosis. *Radiographics* 24:1219-1238, 2004.

Cross-Reference

Thoracic Radiology: THE REQUISITES, 2nd ed, pp 336-337.

Comment

Chronic pulmonary thromboembolism is a relatively uncommon but highly treatable cause of pulmonary artery hypertension. Because many affected patients do not present with a history of prior embolic episodes, the diagnosis may be difficult to make clinically.

Helical CT is playing an increasingly prominent role in the diagnosis of chronic pulmonary thromboembolism. Characteristic findings have been described in the lung parenchyma and pulmonary vessels. With regard to the lung parenchyma, you may observe variable areas of lung attenuation, with a lobular or multilobular distribution, referred to as a mosaic attenuation pattern. In the second figure, note that the low-attenuation areas of the lung have a diminished number and size of vessels compared with adjacent areas of higher attenuation. In patients with chronic pulmonary thromboembolism, this pattern reflects the diminished blood flow to areas of the lung distal to chronic emboli.

The vascular hallmark of chronic pulmonary thromboembolism is the presence of a mural thrombus. Chronic thrombus is typically adherent to the vascular wall, and it may contain foci of calcification. In patients with chronic pulmonary thromboembolism, you may also observe complete occlusion of a vessel that is smaller than its peers; a peripheral intraluminal defect; contrast flowing through thickened, often smaller, arteries due to recanalization; and a web or flap within a contrast-filled artery. In addition, extensive bronchial collateral vessels may also be observed.

Notes

1. What is the reason for complete opacification of the right hemithorax in this young adult man?

2. Name at least four neoplastic causes of an endobronchial lesion.

3. What abnormality is present in the left upper quadrant in the second figure?

4. Name at least one malignant process that can result in an endobronchial lesion and gastric wall thickening.

Complete Lung Collapse Secondary to an Endobronchial Lesion (Lymphoma)

1. Postobstructive atelectasis from an endobronchial lesion.

2. Lung cancer, carcinoid tumor, hamartoma, mucoepidermoid tumor, lymphoma, lipoma, and metastases.

3. Gastric wall thickening.

4. Lymphoma and breast cancer.

Reference

Müller NL, Silva CIS: Atelectasis. In: Silva CIS, Müller NL, Eds. *Imaging of the Chest.* Philadelphia, Saunders, 2008, pp 116-135.

Cross-Reference

Thoracic Radiology: THE REQUISITES, 2nd ed, pp 37, 42.

Comment

Complete opacification of a hemithorax on chest radiography is most commonly caused by complete atelectasis of the underlying lung or by a large ipsilateral pleural effusion. These entities can be readily differentiated by assessing the position of the mediastinum. When atelectasis is the primary abnormality, the mediastinum will be shifted toward the side of opacification. In contrast, when a large pleural effusion is present, the mediastinum will typically be shifted in the opposite direction. In cases of postobstructive atelectasis from an endobronchial lesion, an endobronchial filling defect may be apparent, as seen in the first figure.

Postobstructive atelectasis of an entire lung may occur secondary to a variety of causes. In the intensive care unit (ICU) setting, the presence of an obstructing mucous plug or a malpositioned endotracheal tube (e.g., right mainstem bronchus intubation) should be considered. In an outpatient setting, an obstructing neoplasm or a foreign body (more common in children than in adults) is the most likely etiology. The combination of an endobronchial lesion and gastric wall thickening may occur secondary to lymphoma or breast cancer. Although an endobronchial lesion is a rare manifestation of lymphoma, it is the best choice for the combination of imaging findings in this young adult man.

Notes

1. Name at least two neoplasms that may result in a fine nodular pattern of metastases.

2. Name at least three neoplasms that may result in calcified metastases.

3. Name at least two nonneoplastic causes of a diffuse, fine nodular pattern with calcification.

4. What is the most likely diagnosis in this case?

Metastatic Thyroid Carcinoma

1. Thyroid, melanoma, renal cell carcinoma, and adeno-carcinomas (e.g., breast, pancreas).

2. Thyroid, breast, ovary, colon, sarcomas, and success-fully treated metastases.

3. Healed varicella pneumonia, healed histoplasmosis, silicosis.

4. Metastatic thyroid cancer.

Reference

Reed JC: Diffuse fine nodular opacities. In: *Chest Radiol-ogy: Plain Film Patterns and Differential Diagnoses*, fifth edition. Philadelphia, Mosby, 2003, pp 287-303.

Cross-Reference

Thoracic Radiology: THE REQUISITES, 2nd ed, p 281.

Comment

The radiograph and CT image demonstrate a diffuse, fine nodular pattern of parenchymal opacities. The majority of nodules are 2 to 3 mm in diameter, although a few are slightly larger. The small nodules are well visualized on the radiograph because they are calcified.

Although there are a variety of causes of a fine nodular pattern, only a few entities result in calcified nodules. These entities include healed varicella, healed histoplas-mosis, silicosis, and calcified metastases.

With the exception of osteosarcoma and chondrosar-coma, detectable calcification in metastases is unusual. A variety of mucinous and papillary neoplasms may rarely result in calcified metastases. Thyroid carcinoma is the most common cause of a fine nodular pattern of calcified metastases.

An important ancillary finding in this case is the pres-ence of a superior mediastinal mass, with associated compression and deviation of the trachea. Such masses are usually related to the thyroid gland. In this patient, the mass represents thyroid carcinoma, and the calcified nodules are secondary to metastases.

Notes

1. Name at least one cause of enhancing mediastinal lymph nodes.

2. What neoplasms are typically associated with markedly enhancing mediastinal lymph nodes?

3. Which of the two subtypes of Castleman's disease is more common: hyaline vascular or plasma cell?

4. Which of the two forms is more commonly associated with clinical manifestations?

Castleman's Disease (Benign Lymph Node Hyperplasia)

1. Castleman's disease (angiofollicular lymph node hyperplasia) and hypervascular metastases.

2. Renal cell carcinoma, thyroid cancer, melanoma, and carcinoid neoplasms.

3. Hyaline vascular.

4. Plasma cell.

Reference

Aster JC, Brown JR, Freedman AS: Castleman's disease. In: Rose BD, Ed. *UpToDate*. Waltham, MA, UpToDate, 2009.

Cross-Reference

Thoracic Radiology: THE REQUISITES, 2nd ed, pp 352-353.

Comment

Pregadolinium and postgadolinium coronal MRIs in the first and second figures and a contrast-enhanced CT image in the third figure demonstrate an enhancing nodal mass in the subcarinal region that extends into the azygoesophageal recess. The identification of enhancing nodes significantly narrows the wide differential diagnosis of mediastinal lymph node enlargement. In a majority of cases, enhancing nodes are due to metastatic disease from hypervascular neoplasms such as renal cell, thyroid carcinoma, melanoma, and carcinoid neoplasms. The most common benign etiology is Castleman's disease, the diagnosis in this case, which is an additional important diagnosis to consider when you identify markedly enhancing lymph nodes.

Castleman's disease, also referred to *angiofollicular benign lymph node hyperplasia,* is an uncommon lymphoproliferative disorder. This disorder has been divided into two major histologic subtypes: hyaline vascular and plasma cell. The hyaline vascular subtype is present in the vast majority (90%) of cases. This subtype is characterized by hyperplasia of lymphoid follicles with germinal center formation and the presence of numerous capillaries with hyalinized walls. It usually manifests as a solitary hilar or mediastinal enhancing nodal mass in asymptomatic patients and is generally curable with surgical resection.

The plasma cell subtype is characterized by the presence of mature plasma cells between the hyperplastic germinal centers and relatively few capillaries. This form is frequently associated with clinical symptoms, including fever, fatigue, anemia, polyclonal hypergammaglobulinemia, and bone marrow plasmacytosis. In contrast with the hyaline vascular subtype, bilateral hilar and multifocal mediastinal lymph node enlargement is commonly observed. Another differentiating feature is the relatively low level of enhancement of nodes observed in the plasma cell subtype compared with the marked enhancement of nodes in the hyaline vascular subtype.

Castleman's disease may also be categorized as either unicentric or multicentric in distribution. The former is usually due to the hyaline vascular subtype and the latter is usually secondary to the plasma cell variety. Importantly, multicentric Castleman's disease carries a much worse prognosis than the unicentric variety. Although both varieties may be complicated by development of lymphoma, this is much more common in the multicentric form.

Notes

1. Name at least three substances that are associated with increased signal intensity on T1W MRI.

2. What is the normal appearance of flowing blood within vessels on spin-echo sequences?

3. If this mass is of vascular origin, how can you explain the presence of increased signal intensity?

4. Are spin-echo sequences associated with "black blood" or "white blood" imaging?

Thrombosed Saccular Aortic Aneurysm

1. Fat, hemorrhage (methemoglobin), high protein content, gadolinium, and slow flow in vessels.

2. Signal void (black blood).

3. Thrombosis or slow flow.

4. Black blood.

Reference

Gilkeson RC, Kolodny S: Thoracic aorta. In: Haaga JR, Dogra VS, Forsting M, et al, Eds. *CT and MRI of the Whole Body*, fifth edition. Philadelphia, Elsevier Mosby, 2009, pp 1095-1098.

Cross-Reference

Thoracic Radiology: THE REQUISITES, 2nd ed, pp 358-359.

Comment

The MRI demonstrates a middle mediastinal mass that contacts the lateral aspect of the aortic arch. Whenever you identify a mass immediately adjacent to the aorta, you should always consider an aneurysm. In most cases, the vascular nature of a mass can be readily confirmed by contrast-enhanced CT or MRI.

Vascular imaging with MR historically employed both "black blood" and "white blood" imaging techniques for depiction of aortic anatomy and blood flow, respectively. *Black blood imaging,* as shown in this case, refers to spin-echo sequences. Such sequences result in signal void (black blood) from flowing blood within vascular structures. Although such techniques are excellent for demonstrating the anatomy of vascular structures, including vascular walls and luminal diameter, they are not ideal for assessing luminal flow. In contrast, *white blood techniques* are preferable for assessing luminal flow. There are a variety of white blood techniques, including cine gradient-echo (GRE), two-dimensional segmented time-of-flight, two-dimensional gadolinium-enhanced rapid GRE imaging, and gadolinium-enhanced three-dimensional angiography. These white blood techniques can readily differentiate slow flow from thrombus.

Several newer MRI techniques, including fast imaging with steady-state precession (FISP), optimized k-space filling strategies, parallel imaging techniques, and time-resolved imaging methods, have further improved the ability to assess the aorta using MRI.

This case is challenging. Note the black blood appearance of the aorta in contrast with the increased signal within most of this paraaortic mass. It is important to be aware that slow flow within vascular structures may result in increased signal intensity on T1W images.

An important clue to the diagnosis of this paraaortic mass is the identification of a small, round focus of signal void medially, which connects with the adjacent aortic lumen. Thus, this mass represents a saccular aortic aneurysm. The high signal intensity within the majority of the mass can be explained by either extensive thrombosis or slow flow. A conventional thoracic aortogram confirmed the presence of a thrombosed saccular aortic aneurysm.

Notes

1. In addition to the abnormalities illustrated in these CT images, this patient also had evidence of auricular and nasal abnormalities. What is the most likely cause of airway narrowing?

2. Name at least three additional entities that may be associated with diffuse tracheobronchial narrowing.

3. Which one of these entities characteristically spares the posterior wall of the trachea?

4. Does relapsing polychondritis preferentially involve the proximal or distal airways?

Relapsing Polychondritis

1. Relapsing polychondritis.

2. Tracheopathia osteochondroplastica, Wegener's granulomatosis, amyloidosis, sarcoidosis, infection (papillomatosis, rhinoscleroma, tuberculosis), and saber sheath trachea (associated with COPD).

3. Tracheopathia osteochondroplastica.

4. Proximal.

Reference

Lee KS, Sun MRM, Ernst A, et al: Relapsing polychondritis: prevalence of expiratory CT airway abnormalities. *Radiology* 240:565-573, 2006.

Cross-Reference

Thoracic Radiology: THE REQUISITES, 2nd ed, pp 295, 296.

Comment

The CT images in this case demonstrate diffuse narrowing of the trachea (first figure) and bronchi (second figure), with associated thickening of the tracheal and bronchial walls *(arrows)*. As listed in Answer 2, there are a variety of causes of diffuse tracheobronchial narrowing.

Relapsing polychondritis is a rare inflammatory disease that affects cartilages of the ears, nose, upper respiratory tract, and joints. The etiology of this condition is uncertain, but it is likely an autoimmune disorder. Recurrent bouts of inflammation result in fragmentation and subsequent fibrosis of cartilaginous structures. Auricular chondritis is the most common manifestation of this disorder, occurring in approximately 90% of patients. Respiratory tract involvement is seen in approximately 50% of patients and is the major cause of morbidity associated with this condition.

With regard to airway involvement, the larynx, trachea, and mainstem bronchi are most commonly affected. Segmental and subsegmental bronchi are affected less frequently. Initially, airway narrowing results from mucosal edema. Later in the course of this condition, edema is replaced by granulation tissue and fibrosis. Airway involvement results in impaired clearance of secretions that may be complicated by recurrent respiratory infections and bronchiectasis. Recently, there has been increasing recognition of the presence of tracheobronchomalacia in patients with relapsing polychondritis. This may occur prior to development of morphologic abnormalities in some patients. Thus, imaging evaluation of patients with suspected airway involvement from relapsing polychondritis should include both end-inspiratory and dynamic expiratory sequences.

Dynamic expiratory CT imaging refers to the acquisition of a volumetric CT dataset *during* forced exhalation and has been shown to be more sensitive for detecting malacia than the less physiologic method of end-expiratory imaging.

Notes

1. Name the syndrome characterized by a unilateral hyperlucent lung or lobe secondary to an obliterative bronchiolitis (OB).

2. What is the cause of this syndrome?

3. What methods can be used to demonstrate air trapping in patients with this condition?

4. What airway abnormality is frequently demonstrated on CT scans of patients with this syndrome?

Swyer-James Syndrome

1. Swyer-James syndrome (also known as MacLeod syndrome).

2. Acute viral bronchiolitis in infancy or childhood.

3. Expiratory radiograph or CT and nuclear medicine ventilation scan.

4. Bronchiectasis.

Reference

Silva CT, Müller NL: Broncholitis. In: Müller NL, Silva CI, Eds. *Imaging of the Chest.* Philadelphia, Saunders, 2008, pp 1090-1092.

Cross-Reference

Thoracic Radiology: THE REQUISITES, 2nd ed, pp 324, 325.

Comment

The chest radiograph demonstrates hyperlucency of the left lung with associated reduced pulmonary vascularity, which is most marked in the left lower lobe. Also note the slightly reduced size of the left lung compared with the right lung.

The imaging findings are characteristic of Swyer-James syndrome, a variant of postinfectious OB. This syndrome occurs secondary to an acute viral bronchiolitis in early infancy or early childhood that prevents the normal development of the affected lung. As shown in this case, the typical inspiratory radiograph findings include a unilateral hyperlucent lung or lobe with normal or reduced volume and reduced pulmonary vascularity. Expiratory radiographs (not shown) reveal air trapping.

HRCT imaging features of Swyer-James syndrome include (1) areas of decreased lung attenuation with associated reduction in the number and size of vessels; (2) bronchiectasis; and (3) air trapping on expiratory images. Interestingly, although radiographic findings in patients with Swyer-James syndrome are typically unilateral, CT scanning often shows patchy areas of abnormality within the opposite lung as well.

Most patients are asymptomatic adults at the time of diagnosis, and the condition is often detected incidentally on a radiograph or CT performed for other reasons. Less commonly, patients present with recurrent infections or dyspnea.

Notes

1. What is the most likely cause for the bronchiectasis and centrilobular nodules in this elderly woman who presents with a chronic cough?

2. Is this the classic form of *Mycobacterium avium* complex (MAC) infection?

3. Is bronchopulmonary MAC infection acquired by human-to-human transmission?

4. In older women with MAC infection, which lobes of the lungs are most frequently affected?

Mycobacterium avium Complex (MAC) Infection

1. MAC infection.

2. No.

3. No.

4. Middle lobe and lingula.

Reference

Erasmus JJ, McAdams HP, Farrell MA, Patz EF Jr: Pulmonary nontuberculous mycobacterial infection: radiologic manifestations. *Radiographics* 19:1487-1505, 1999.

Cross-Reference

Thoracic Radiology: THE REQUISITES, 2nd ed, pp 105-107.

Comment

Nontuberculous mycobacterial (NTMB) infection is usually caused by MAC and *Mycobacterium kansasii.* These organisms are found in soil and water and demonstrate similar features.

NTMB affects two main groups of patients, who present with distinct demographic, clinical, and radiographic features. The first group consists primarily of older men with COPD. Such patients present with the classic form of NTMB infection, which may occur secondary to either MAC or *M. kansasii.* Clinical symptoms are often insidious and include cough, hemoptysis, and constitutional symptoms. The imaging features are almost identical to those of reactivation TB and are characterized by slowly progressive fibronodular opacities that are often associated with cavitation. The apical and posterior segments of the upper lobes and the superior segments of the lower lobes are most commonly involved.

The second group of patients is composed of elderly women with MAC infection. Such patients are immunocompetent and do not have a history of COPD. They typically present with chronic cough, but hemoptysis and constitutional symptoms are usually absent. The imaging features of MAC in this subgroup are best demonstrated by CT and include cylindrical bronchiectasis and multiple small (usually less than 5-mm-diameter) centrilobular nodules and/or tree-in-bud opacities. Foci of ground-glass opacification and consolidation may also be encountered. In contrast with the classic form of MAC infection, cavitation is uncommon in this subgroup. Although the distribution may be diffuse, the middle lobe and lingula are most commonly involved.

Because NTMB are common contaminants in the human environment, a diagnosis requires (1) evidence of cavitation or progressive changes on chest radiographs (classic form); (2) at least two positive sputum cultures; or (3) evidence of mycobacteria on biopsy or BAL. Precise identification of the infecting organism is important for directing appropriate therapy.

Notes

1. What is the term used to describe this bronchial abnormality?

2. Is this a congenital or an acquired condition?

3. From what portion of the airway does it arise?

4. Name at least one symptom associated with this condition.

Cardiac Bronchus

1. Cardiac bronchus.

2. Congenital.

3. Bronchus intermedius.

4. Recurrent infections, hemoptysis, cough, and dyspnea.

Reference

McGuinness G, Naidich DP, Garay SM, et al: Accessory cardiac bronchus: CT features and clinical significance. *Radiology* 189:563-566, 1993.

Cross-Reference

Thoracic Radiology: THE REQUISITES, 2nd ed, pp 306-307.

Comment

The CT image in this case demonstrates an anomalous blind-ending diverticulum *(arrow)* arising from the medial wall of the bronchus intermedius. This structure represents a cardiac bronchus, the only known true supernumerary anomalous bronchus. Other anomalies of the airway involve either a normal number of bronchi with ectopic locations (e.g., aberrant tracheal bronchus) or an absence of bronchi (e.g., bronchial atresia).

The cardiac bronchus always arises from the same location—the medial wall of the bronchus intermedius, above the origin of the superior segment bronchus. It is directed caudally toward the mediastinum. For this reason, it has been coined the *cardiac* bronchus.

Its length varies from a small, blind-ending pouch (such as in this case) to a longer branching structure. The longer configuration may be associated with rudimentary alveolar tissue in some cases. The cardiac bronchus is lined by endobronchial mucosa and contains cartilaginous rings within its walls.

This anomaly is usually incidentally discovered in asymptomatic patients. However, because a cardiac bronchus may serve as a reservoir for infectious material, affected patients may present with recurrent respiratory infections. Resultant inflammation and hypervascularity may also result in hemoptysis. Surgical excision is recommended for symptomatic patients.

Notes

1. What congenital vascular abnormality is present?

2. What is the prevalence of this anomaly?

3. What is the term used to describe the swallowing difficulty associated with this anomaly?

4. What acquired aortic abnormality is also present in this case?

Aberrant Right Subclavian Artery With Aortic Dissection

1. Aberrant right subclavian artery.

2. Approximately 1%.

3. Dysphagia lusoria.

4. Aortic dissection.

Reference

Freed K, Low VHS: The aberrant subclavian artery. *AJR Am J Roentgenol* 166:481-484, 1997.

Cross-Reference

Thoracic Radiology: THE REQUISITES, 2nd ed, pp 355-356.

Comment

An *aberrant right subclavian artery (ARSA)* is the most common intrathoracic major arterial anomaly, with an incidence of approximately 1%. The ARSA arises as the last branch of the aortic arch and courses cephalad obliquely from left to right behind the trachea and esophagus. An aortic diverticulum, the diverticulum of Kommerell, may be present at the origin of this vessel.

In most patients, the anomaly is asymptomatic and discovered incidentally. A small minority of patients may develop difficulty in swallowing secondary to esophageal compression.

On chest radiography, you may observe the ARSA as an oblique opacity coursing superiorly from left to right, beginning at the level of the aortic arch. On barium swallow examinations, you may observe a characteristic oblique indentation on the posterior wall of the esophagus. An ARSA is easily identified on cross-sectional imaging studies such as the CT images in the figures. On such studies, the ARSA appears as a tubular structure arising from the aortic arch and coursing cephalad obliquely behind the trachea and esophagus. Aneurysmal dilation of the proximal portion of the ARSA is observed in approximately 10% of cases.

This case also demonstrates the presence of an aortic dissection. Note the presence of an intimal flap, which appears as a linear soft tissue density within the contrast-opacified vessels. Aortic dissection is characterized by a tear in the intima of the aortic wall, followed by separation of the tunica media. This process results in the creation of two channels for the passage of blood: a true and a false lumen.

Once you have identified an aortic dissection, it is important to determine its precise extent. Involvement of the ascending aorta (Stanford type A) requires surgical therapy. Extension of the dissection into the great vessels is an important preoperative finding. In contrast, isolated descending aortic dissections (Stanford type B) are generally managed medically.

Notes

A

B

1. What is the most common source of arterial blood supply for a sequestration?

2. Which form of sequestration is more common, intralobar or extralobar?

3. Are sequestrations more common in the left or the right lung?

4. What is the usual drainage site for an intralobar sequestration?

Intralobar Sequestration

1. Descending thoracic aorta.

2. Intralobar.

3. Left.

4. Inferior pulmonary vein.

Reference

Lee EY, Boiselle PM, Cleveland RH: Evaluation of congenital lung anomalies. *Radiology* 247:632-648, 2008.

Cross-Reference

Thoracic Radiology: THE REQUISITES, 2nd ed, pp 68-70.

Comment

The chest radiograph demonstrates a focal opacity in the posterior basal segment of the left lower lobe, which obscures a portion of the descending thoracic aortic interface and medial left hemidiaphragm. The CT image reveals a discrete soft tissue density mass that contains two tiny cystic foci. Note the presence of an adjacent tubular structure *(arrow)*, which represents a systemic artery from the descending thoracic aorta. The imaging findings are consistent with a *sequestration,* which refers to an area of aberrant lung tissue that has no normal connection with the bronchial tree or pulmonary arteries and is supplied by a systemic artery.

Sequestrations are classified as either *intralobar* (contained within the substance of the lung) or *extralobar* (contained within its own pleural envelope). Intralobar sequestration is the most common type. Affected patients may be asymptomatic or may present with a history of recurrent pulmonary infections. The posterior basal segment is the most common location, and the left lung is affected twice as often as the right lung. Intralobar sequestrations may appear radiographically as a solid mass, a focal area of consolidation, or a cystic or multicystic lesion. The identification of a systemic arterial supply confirms the diagnosis. A systemic artery is usually visible on either contrast-enhanced CT or MRI. Failure to detect such a vessel does not exclude the diagnosis, however, and angiography may rarely be required for definitive diagnosis.

In contrast with intralobar sequestration, the extralobar variety usually presents during infancy. The typical radiographic appearance is a well-defined, solitary mass in close proximity to the posteromedial aspect of the hemidiaphragm. Less frequent sites of involvement include mediastinal and subdiaphragmatic locations. Approximately 90% of cases are in the left hemithorax. The arterial supply may arise from single or multiple systemic arteries. Extralobar sequestration is associated with systemic venous drainage, usually to the azygos system and less commonly into the portal vein, subclavian vein, or internal mammary vein.

Whereas extralobar sequestration is widely recognized as a congenital anomaly, there is emerging consensus that intralobar sequestration may be acquired secondary to chronic infection.

Notes

1. This patient is status post transplantation of the left lung 2 weeks prior to the date of these radiographs, which were obtained 2 days apart. Considering this time interval, is reperfusion edema (reimplantation response) a likely diagnosis?

2. Are pleural effusions a common finding in patients with acute rejection?

3. Does a normal chest radiograph exclude the presence of acute rejection?

4. On what basis is a diagnosis of acute rejection typically made?

Acute Rejection Following Lung Transplantation

1. No.

2. Yes.

3. No.

4. Histologic analysis of transbronchial biopsy specimens.

Reference

Erasmus JJ, McAdams HP, Tapson VF, et al: Radiologic issues in lung transplantation for end-stage pulmonary disease. *AJR Am J Roentgenol* 169:69-78, 1997.

Cross-Reference

None.

Comment

Lung transplantation is a potentially life-saving therapeutic option for certain patients with end-stage pulmonary disease. Because of the limited supply of donor lungs, single- rather than double-lung transplantation is usually performed. Single-lung transplantation is also technically easier to perform and has a slightly lower morbidity and mortality than double-lung transplantation. Most pulmonary disorders, including various causes of pulmonary fibrosis and emphysema, can be successfully managed with single-lung transplantation. Exceptions are disorders such as cystic fibrosis that are associated with chronically infected lungs. Such patients require double-lung transplantation. Recently, transplantation of lobes from living-related donors has also been performed in patients with cystic fibrosis.

Early pulmonary postoperative complications of lung transplantation include reperfusion edema, acute rejection, and infection. *Reperfusion edema,* also referred to as *reimplantation response,* is caused by increased capillary permeability and occurs in the vast majority of transplanted lungs. It has a characteristic time course, usually beginning in the first 24 hours, peaking between 1 and 5 days, and resolving within approximately 10 days following transplantation. Acute rejection is a common complication within the first 3 months following transplantation. The first episode usually occurs in the first 5 to 10 days following surgery. Note that reperfusion edema begins earlier and peaks before this time. Infection is the most common pulmonary complication following transplantation. The type of organism varies depending on the time interval from surgery. In the first month, bacterial infections are most common. After the first month, atypical infections such as cytomegalovirus (CMV) are most common.

Notes

1. What is the most likely mechanism for involvement of the airways by TB in this case?

2. Are the imaging features suggestive of the hyperplastic or the fibrostenotic stage of TB airway involvement?

3. Is the hyperplastic form of tuberculous airways disease potentially reversible with therapy?

4. Are these imaging findings specific for an infectious process?

TB Involving the Airways

1. Direct invasion from adjacent mediastinal lymph nodes.

2. Hyperplastic.

3. Yes.

4. No—neoplasm should be excluded.

References

Jeong YJ, Lee KS: Pulmonary tuberculosis: up-to-date imaging and management. *AJR Am J Roentgenol* 191:834-844, 2008.

Moon WK, Mim J, Yeon KM, Han MC: Tuberculosis of the central airways: CT findings of active and fibrotic disease. *AJR Am J Roentgenol* 169:648-653, 1997.

Cross-Reference

Thoracic Radiology: THE REQUISITES, 2nd ed, pp 299, 300.

Comment

Airway involvement has been reported in 10% to 20% of all patients with pulmonary TB. It may result from several mechanisms: (1) direct contact of the airway mucosa with infected secretions; (2) submucosal spread of infection through the lymphatics from infected lymph nodes or lung; and (3) direct invasion of the airway by adjacent lymph nodes.

There are two stages of tracheobronchial involvement by TB. The first stage is characterized by hyperplastic changes. During this stage, tubercles form in the submucosal layer and are accompanied by ulceration and necrosis of the airway wall. The affected airway walls appear irregularly thickened with variable degrees of luminal narrowing. Hilar and mediastinal lymph node enlargement are commonly observed and frequently demonstrate peripheral enhancement with central low attenuation. Cavitary lung lesions may occasionally be seen within the lobes drained by the affected bronchi.

In the first figure, note the presence of irregular thickening of the anterior and lateral wall of the trachea, with eccentric luminal narrowing. In the second figure, there is irregular, lobulated thickening of the anterior wall of the airway with polypoid intraluminal extension. The contiguity of the airway disease with adjacent mediastinal lymph nodes suggests that the airway involvement is due to direct invasion by tuberculous lymph nodes.

The second stage is characterized by fibrostenotic features. In this stage, the bronchi are typically smoothly narrowed. The fibrostenotic phase can be complicated by postobstructive collapse.

In a study of 41 patients with TB of the airway, patients with a hyperplastic stage of TB demonstrated irregular and thick-walled airways, a pattern frequently reversible with medical therapy. In contrast, patients with fibrotic disease generally demonstrated smooth narrowing of the airways and minimal wall thickening, a pattern not reversible with medical therapy.

Notes

1. Name three disease entities that may manifest on CT as diffuse ground-glass opacity.

2. On thin-section CT, what distinguishes ground-glass opacity from consolidation?

3. Name the seven idiopathic interstitial pneumonias recognized by the American Thoracic Society (ATS) and the European Respiratory Society (ERS).

4. Which interstitial lung diseases may manifest on thin-section CT as the usual interstitial pneumonia (UIP) pattern?

CASE 138

Acute Interstitial Pneumonia (AIP)

1. Pulmonary edema, pulmonary hemorrhage, hypersensitivity pneumonitis, atypical infections (*Pneumocystis jiroveci* pneumonia, CMV pneumonia)

2. Ground-glass opacity does not obscure underlying lung structures; consolidation does obscure those structures.

3. Idiopathic pulmonary fibrosis (IPF), nonspecific interstitial pneumonia (NSIP), cryptogenic organizing pneumonia (COP), acute interstitial pneumonia (AIP), respiratory bronchiolitis–interstitial lung (RB-ILD), desquamative interstitial pneumonia (DIP), and lymphocytic interstitial pneumonia (LIP).

4. Idiopathic pulmonary fibrosis (IPF), connective tissue diseases (rheumatoid arthritis, scleroderma), asbestosis, and drug-related lung injury (e.g., bleomycin toxicity).

Reference

Johkoh T, Müller NL, Taniguchi H, et al: Acute interstitial pneumonia: thin-section CT findings in 36 patients. *Radiology* 211:859-863, 1999.

Cross-Reference

Thoracic Radiology: THE REQUISITES, 2nd ed, pp 194, 195.

Comment

AIP is a rapidly progressive form of lung injury that represents an idiopathic form of adult respiratory distress syndrome (ARDS) and diffuse alveolar damage (DAD). A diffuse interstitial pneumonia that was originally thought to represent a rapidly progressive form of UIP, AIP is now recognized as a separate clinicopathologic entity and occurs much less commonly than UIP.

The diffuse idiopathic interstitial pneumonias (IIPs) have distinct clinical manifestations, pathologic features, and imaging findings and were classified in 2001 by an international consensus statement issued by the ATS and the ERS that recognized seven distinct clinicopathologic entities: IPF (UIP), NSIP, COP, AIP, RB-ILD, DIP, and LIP. Diffuse parenchymal diseases due to known causes and associations such as drugs and connective tissue diseases are not considered idiopathic.

Notes

1. Name at least one cardiogenic cause of pulmonary edema associated with pregnancy.

2. Name at least one noncardiogenic cause of pulmonary edema associated with pregnancy.

3. Is pregnancy associated with an increased prevalence of pulmonary thromboembolic disease?

4. Why are pregnant patients at increased risk for community-acquired pneumonias?

Pregnancy Complicated by Pulmonary Edema Secondary to Preeclampsia

1. Peripartum cardiomyopathy and hypertension (preeclampsia).

2. Tocolytic therapy and amniotic fluid embolism.

3. Yes.

4. Pregnancy is associated with a depression in cell-mediated immunity.

Reference

Fidler JL, Patz EF, Ravin CE: Cardiopulmonary complications of pregnancy: radiographic findings. *AJR Am J Roentgenol* 161:937-941, 1993.

Cross-Reference

None.

Comment

Pregnancy is normally associated with a variety of cardiopulmonary physiologic changes. Maternal blood volume and cardiac output increase by approximately 45% by midpregnancy. These changes are associated with increased pulmonary vascularity and progressive left ventricular dilation and mild hypertrophy.

There are a variety of cardiopulmonary complications of pregnancy, including cardiogenic and noncardiogenic pulmonary edema, pulmonary thromboembolism, aspiration pneumonitis, and pneumonia. Other rare complications include metastatic disease from gestational trophoblastic neoplasm, pneumothorax, and pneumomediastinum.

The patient in this case developed preeclampsia during her third trimester of pregnancy that was complicated by pulmonary edema. Preeclampsia is characterized by the development of hypertension, proteinuria, and edema after 24 weeks' gestation. *Eclampsia* refers to the development of seizures. In patients with preeclampsia, hypertension may become severe enough to produce acute cardiac failure. Radiographs typically show pulmonary edema with a variable heart size. In this patient, the pulmonary edema was asymmetric, reflecting gravitational dependency of pulmonary edema due to the patient's preference for lying on her left side. Another cardiogenic cause of pulmonary edema is peripartum cardiomyopathy, which occurs in the last month of pregnancy or in the first 6 months following delivery. Radiographs demonstrate marked cardiac enlargement that may be accompanied by pulmonary edema.

Notes

1. What term is used to describe the fat attenuation mass located in the interatrial septum in the figure?

2. Is this a benign or malignant process?

3. In what percentage of cases is this process associated with diffuse mediastinal lipomatosis?

4. Does this entity typically enhance following intravenous contrast administration?

Lipomatous Hypertrophy of the Interatrial Septum (LHIS)

1. LHIS.

2. Benign.

3. Approximately 50%.

4. No.

Reference

Fan CM, Fischman AJ, Kewk BH, et al: Lipomatous hypertrophy of the interatrial septum: increased uptake on FDG PET. *AJR Am J Roentgenol* 184:339-342, 2005.

Cross-Reference

None.

Comment

LHIS refers to the presence of a fat-attenuation interatrial mass. LHIS is usually incidentally detected on CT scans of asymptomatic patients. An association with atrial arrhythmias has been reported in some cases and is thought to occur secondary to disruption of septal conduction pathways.

Pathologically, LHIS demonstrates multiloculated, granular lipocytes within the interatrial septum. In contrast to lipomas, the adipose tissue in LHIS is unencapsulated. The lipocytes in LHIS are the morphologic cells found in fetal or brown fat. Interestingly, LHIS may result in false-positive findings on PET scans due to preferential uptake of 2-[fluorine-18] fluoro-2-deoxy-D-glucose (FDG) by brown fat, especially in the fasting state. Thus, when you see increased uptake within the right heart on FDG-PET studies, you should carefully correlate with CT findings for the presence of LHIS to avoid a false-positive diagnosis of cardiac malignancy.

The typical CT appearance is a nonenhancing, smoothly marginated, dumbbell-shaped, homogeneous, fat attenuation mass that is usually confined to the interatrial septum. The characteristic dumbbell shape is due to sparing of the fossa ovalis.

Notes

1. What is the striking abnormality on this MR angiogram?

2. Is a unilateral central pulmonary embolus (PE) a common distribution of acute pulmonary thromboembolism?

3. What is the radiographic sign used to describe oligemia distal to an obstructing embolus?

4. On MRI, how can you differentiate a pulmonary artery sarcoma from an acute thrombus?

Massive Unilateral PE

1. Abrupt cutoff of the left main pulmonary artery (LPA).

2. No.

3. Westermark's sign.

4. Only a pulmonary artery sarcoma enhances with gadolinium.

Reference
Remy-Jardin M, Pistolesi M, Goodman LR, et al: Management of suspected acute pulmonary embolism in the era of CT angiography: a statement from the Fleischner Society. *Radiology* 245:315-329, 2007.

Cross-Reference
Thoracic Radiology: THE REQUISITES, 2nd ed, pp 332-336.

Comment
The MR angiogram demonstrates a normal appearance of the pulmonary vasculature of the right lung and complete absence of pulmonary vasculature within the left lung. Note the abrupt cut-off of the LPA due to an acute embolus.

A unilateral, completely obstructing embolus is an uncommon manifestation of acute pulmonary thromboembolism. In fact, when confronted with a nuclear medicine ventilation-perfusion scan that demonstrates a unilateral absence of perfusion, you should first consider nonthromboembolic causes such as mediastinal and hilar masses, ascending aortic aneurysm and dissection, pulmonary artery hypoplasia and agenesis, and pulmonary artery sarcoma and pneumonectomy. In this patient, the MRI examination revealed an obstructing, nonenhancing intrinsic filling defect in the LPA, consistent with an acute PE.

Several exciting recent technologic advances in MRI, including parallel imaging, view sharing, and time-resolved echo-shared angiography techniques, have resulted in an enhanced ability to evaluate for PE with MRI owing to shortened acquisition times, reduced motion artifacts, and improved spatial resolution.

According to the 2007 Fleischner Society statement regarding management of suspected acute PE, MR angiography of the pulmonary arteries and MR venography for deep vein thrombosis performed with state-of-the-art techniques can potentially serve as a second-line examination in the evaluation of suspected acute PE in patients who are unable to receive iodinated contrast material for CT or for whom ionizing radiation is of concern. Currently, CT angiography remains the study of choice for acute PE owing to its high accuracy, widespread access, rapid acquisition time, and superb ability to simultaneously assess the lungs for potential alternative diagnoses.

Notes

1. What disorder is most closely associated with a basilar distribution of panlobular emphysema?

2. Is there any association between this entity and bronchiectasis?

3. How is this disorder inherited?

4. Name an abdominal complication of this disorder.

C A S E 1 4 2

Alpha$_1$-antitrypsin (AAT) Deficiency

1. AAT deficiency.

2. Yes.

3. Autosomal recessive.

4. Cirrhosis.

Reference
Wood AM, Stockley RA: Alpha one antitrypsin deficiency: from gene to treatment. *Respiration* 74:481-492, 2007.

Cross-Reference
Thoracic Radiology: THE REQUISITES, 2nd ed, pp 244-245.

Comment
The CT image demonstrates diffuse panlobular emphysema in the lower lung zones. The upper lobes (not shown) were relatively spared of this process. *Panlobular emphysema* is characterized by fewer and smaller-than-normal pulmonary vessels. This appearance has been described as a *simplification of normal lung architecture.* AAT deficiency, the diagnosis in this case, is characterized by a basilar distribution of panlobular emphysema.

   AAT deficiency, also referred to as *alpha$_1$-protease inhibitor deficiency,* is an inherited disorder that is characterized by abnormally low levels of alpha$_1$-protease inhibitor. This protein inhibits a number of lysosomal proteases and prevents the damaging effects of elastases released by macrophages and neutrophils. Because the administration of elastase has been shown to produce emphysema in animal models, it is not surprising that patients with reduced levels of protease inhibitors are at risk for developing this complication. Patients who are homozygous for this disorder have a very low level (approximately 20% of normal) of alpha$_1$-protease inhibitor and are at high risk for developing emphysema. This risk is increased by cigarette smoking.

   Interestingly, patients with AAT deficiency have a high prevalence of bronchiectasis, which has been reported in approximately 40% of cases. In the figure, note the presence of bronchial wall thickening and dilation, which is most pronounced in the right lower lobe. The mechanism by which bronchiectasis develops in these patients is uncertain. It has been hypothesized that destruction of elastic fibers in the walls of bronchi and bronchioles plays an important role in this process.

   Treatment approaches targeting the molecular basis of this disease are currently under investigation and include AAT replacement, gene therapy, and stem cells.

Notes

1. What is the predominant distribution of the parenchymal opacities shown in these CT images?

2. In contrast, what is the distribution of the focal right middle lobe consolidation shown in the second image?

3. Name at least three entities that typically present with a peripheral pattern of consolidation.

4. Which of these entities frequently demonstrates both peripheral and peribronchovascular foci of consolidation on CT imaging?

Cryptogenic Organizing Pneumonia

1. Peripheral.

2. Peribronchovascular.

3. COP, Löffler's syndrome, chronic eosinophilic pneumonia, pulmonary infarcts, and vasculitides.

4. COP.

Reference

Mueller-Mang C, Grosse C, Schmid K, et al: What every radiologist should know about idiopathic interstitial pneumonias. *Radiographics* 27:595-615, 2007.

Cross-Reference

Thoracic Radiology: THE REQUISITES, 2nd ed, pp 199-200.

Comment

Organizing pneumonia is characterized pathologically by the presence of granulation tissue polyps within the alveolar ducts and alveoli. Although it may be idiopathic, organizing pneumonia has been described in association with a number of entities, including pulmonary infection, drug reactions, collagen-vascular disorders, and vasculitides. Thus, the diagnosis of COP requires the exclusion of known underlying causes.

Affected patients typically present clinically with a nonproductive cough. Associated symptoms may include dyspnea, malaise, and low-grade fever. The majority of cases respond to steroids and have a favorable prognosis. However, some patients relapse following cessation of therapy. Interestingly, lung parenchymal opacities associated with COP may migrate, even in the absence of treatment.

Radiographic findings consist primarily of patchy, nonsegmental, unilateral or bilateral foci of consolidation. The characteristic peripheral distribution of consolidation associated with COP may not be readily apparent on chest radiographs and is seen more frequently on CT scans.

Characteristic HRCT imaging features include patchy bilateral airspace consolidation with a peripheral or peribronchovascular distribution. In some cases, the extreme subpleural region of the lung is spared. The opacities may vary from ground glass to consolidation. In some cases, the periphery may appear more dense than the center, an appearance referred to as the *reverse halo* or *atoll sign.* Poorly defined lung nodules may also be observed and are often peribronchiolar in distribution. Thus, the presence of peripheral and peribronchovascular consolidation with associated small lung nodules in this case is most suggestive of COP.

Notes

1. Name at least four indications for tracheobronchial stent placement.

2. List at least four potential complications of airway stent placement.

3. What complication is evident in this case?

4. Are metallic airway stents easily removable?

Fractured Tracheal Stent

1. Anastomotic narrowing following lung transplantation; palliative treatment of unresectable malignancy involving the trachea or bronchi; congenital or acquired tracheal stenosis; tracheobronchomalacia; external tracheal compression; and tracheal narrowing due to inflammatory or infectious etiologies.

2. Airway inflammation; stent migration; airway erosion; stent fracture; intraluminal narrowing due to granulation tissue; stent collapse; tracheoesophageal fistula; tracheobronchial perforation; and invasion by adjacent neoplasm.

3. Stent fracture.

4. No.

Reference
Dialani V, Ernst A, Sun M, et al: MDCT detection of airway stent complications: comparison with bronchoscopy. *AJR Am J Roentgenol* 191:1576-1580, 2008.

Cross-Reference
None.

Comment
The axial CT image in the first figure and the two-dimensional sagittal reformatted image in the second figure demonstrate the presence of a tracheal stent within the lower cervical portion of the trachea. Note the presence of focal stent fracture and disruption posteriorly *(arrows)*. This patient underwent stent placement for tracheal stenosis. She subsequently presented with evidence of wire fragments in her sputum, prompting this CT examination.

Airway stents are increasingly employed in the treatment of a variety of airway abnormalities. There are two major types: metallic and silicone. Once placed into the airway, metallic stents become incorporated into the bronchial wall or epithelialized, limiting potential migration and permitting ciliary activity to continue. Metallic stents are difficult to remove once employed and have a greater complication rate than silicone stents. For this reason, their use should be limited to palliative treatment of patients with inoperable airway involvement by malignancy. Patients with airway compromise due to benign causes should be treated with silicone stents.

Prior to the advent of airway stenting, the treatment of tracheal stenosis was limited to surgical therapy. Surgical treatment of tracheal abnormalities with end-to-end reanastomosis is possible only when there is sufficient length of the airway. Stenting is not limited by this factor and thus provides an additional therapeutic option for many patients who are not surgical candidates.

Prior to stent placement, CT accurately depicts the number and length of airway stenoses. Following placement of a stent, CT is an ideal modality for assessing for complications such as stent migration, stent fracture, and intraluminal narrowing. Recently, MDCT has been shown to be highly accurate for detecting stent complications, with similar accuracy to the reference standard of bronchoscopy.

Notes

1. What is the most likely cause of this completely cystic anterior mediastinal mass?

2. Name at least two etiologies for an anterior mediastinal mass that contains solid and cystic elements.

3. What is the most common cause of a thymic mass?

4. If a thymic cyst has been complicated by hemorrhage, how would you expect it to appear on T1W MRI?

Thymic Cyst

1. Thymic cyst.

2. Thymoma, germ cell neoplasms, and Hodgkin's disease (uncommon manifestation).

3. Thymoma.

4. Bright (hemorrhage results in increased signal on T1W images as a result of the T1 shortening effect of methemoglobin).

Reference

Jeung MY, Gasser B, Gangi A, et al: Imaging of cystic masses of the mediastinum. *Radiographics* 22:S79-S93, 2002.

Cross-Reference

Thoracic Radiology: THE REQUISITES, 2nd ed, p 349.

Comment

Thymic cysts are an uncommon cause of an anterior mediastinal mass. They may be congenital or acquired. Congenital cysts are probably derived from remnants of the fetal thymopharyngeal duct. Acquired cysts may develop following radiation therapy for Hodgkin's disease. Less commonly, they may occur following thoracotomy or after chemotherapy for a malignant neoplasm. An association with human immunodeficiency virus (HIV) infection has also been reported.

On imaging studies, a thymic cyst typically appears as a well-defined, cystic mass with an imperceptible wall. In a minority of cases, curvilinear calcifications may be identified within the wall of thymic cysts. On CT, thymic cysts typically demonstrate fluid attenuation. On MRI, thymic cysts usually demonstrate low signal intensity on T1W images and increased signal intensity on T2W images. However, the appearance may vary if the cyst has been complicated by hemorrhage or infection. The imaging features in this case are typical of an uncomplicated thymic cyst. Incidentally noted are numerous calcified pleural plaques, consistent with prior asbestos exposure.

When you identify an anterior mediastinal mass with solid and cystic components, you should consider the possibility of a solid anterior mediastinal mass that has undergone cystic necrosis. For example, thymoma and Hodgkin's lymphoma may contain cystic areas, occasionally associated with a relatively small amount of neoplastic tissue. Germ cell neoplasms such as mature teratomas frequently contain cystic components intermixed with solid elements. The identification of cystic elements in conjunction with fat and/or calcium should suggest this diagnosis.

Notes

1. What congenital airway abnormality is evident on the three-dimensional reconstruction image of the trachea?

2. What portion of the lung does this anomalous bronchus usually supply?

3. Are patients with this finding usually symptomatic?

4. What potential complication can occur following intubation of a patient with this abnormality?

Tracheal Bronchus

1. Tracheal bronchus.

2. Right upper lobe (apical segment or entire lobe).

3. No.

4. Atelectasis of the portion of the lung supplied by the anomalous bronchus.

Reference

Ghaye B, Szapiro D, Fanchamps JM, Dondelinger RF: Congenital bronchial abnormalities revisited. *Radiographics* 21:105-119, 2001.

Cross-Reference

Thoracic Radiology: THE REQUISITES, 2nd ed, pp 59, 62.

Comment

The tomogram demonstrates an anomalous bronchus arising from the right lateral wall of the trachea, proximal to the origin of the right mainstem bronchus. The term *tracheal bronchus* has been used to describe this congenital bronchial anomaly, which may supply the apical segment of the right upper lobe or the entire right upper lobe. The latter configuration is also referred to as a *pig bronchus.*

Affected patients are usually asymptomatic. In a minority of cases, the bronchial orifice is narrow, which may lead to recurrent pneumonias and bronchiectasis. Following intubation, the aberrant bronchus may become occluded by the endotracheal tube balloon cuff, resulting in atelectasis within the corresponding segment or lobe that is supplied by the aberrant bronchus.

Notes

1. What is striking about these pulmonary nodules on this noncontrast CT?

2. Considering the presence of a hyperdense liver, what is the most likely etiology for these nodules?

3. What disorder is amiodarone used to treat?

4. What percentage of patients treated with amiodarone develop pulmonary toxicity?

Amiodarone Drug Toxicity

1. High attenuation.

2. Amiodarone toxicity.

3. Arrhythmias.

4. Approximately 5% to 20%.

Reference

Rossi SE, Erasmus JJ, McAdams HP, et al: Pulmonary drug toxicity: radiologic and pathologic manifestations. *Radiographics* 20:1245-1259, 2000.

Cross-Reference

Thoracic Radiology: THE REQUISITES, 2nd ed, pp 234, 235.

Comment

The noncontrast CT images presented in this case demonstrate several small pulmonary nodules with a subpleural distribution. Note the high attenuation of these lesions, a finding that is characteristic of lung toxicity due to amiodarone, a triiodinated compound that is used to treat cardiac arrhythmias. Pulmonary toxicity occurs in 5% to 20% of patients treated with amiodarone and is dose related.

There are three distinct clinical presentations of amiodarone toxicity. The most common presentation is a subacute onset of dyspnea, nonproductive cough, and weight loss. Radiographs typically reveal a diffuse linear pattern that may be difficult to distinguish from congestive heart failure. This usually correlates pathologically with an NSIP pattern. A less common presentation (observed in approximately one third of patients) is characterized by an acute onset of symptoms that mimic an infectious pneumonitis. Radiographs of these patients typically demonstrate patchy alveolar opacities with a peripheral distribution that correlate pathologically with COP. Unenhanced CT scans in these patients typically reveal high-attenuation foci of parenchymal opacification, with attenuation values ranging from approximately 80 to 175 Hounsfield units. This appearance reflects the high concentration of amiodarone, a triiodinated agent, within these regions of lung parenchyma. A third rare but potentially fatal form of pulmonary toxicity is ARDS.

Note the high attenuation of the liver in the second figure, a common finding in patients treated with amiodarone. Thus, the combination of high-attenuation focal parenchymal opacities and a high-attenuation liver is highly suggestive of amiodarone pulmonary toxicity. Prompt recognition is important, because amiodarone pulmonary toxicity is frequently reversible after withdrawal of the drug. Although clinical symptoms usually resolve within 2 to 4 weeks of drug withdrawal, chest radiographic abnormalities typically clear more slowly, in approximately 3 months.

Notes

1. What is the predominant distribution of nodules shown in these HRCT images?

2. Name at least three entities that can be associated with this distribution.

3. Which of these entities is frequently associated with symmetric hilar lymph node enlargement?

4. Is air trapping a frequent observation on expiratory CT images of patients with sarcoidosis?

Sarcoidosis

1. Axial (peribronchovascular).

2. Sarcoidosis, lymphangitic carcinomatosis, lymphoma, and Kaposi's sarcoma.

3. Sarcoidosis.

4. Yes.

Reference

Koyama T, Ueda H, Togashi K, et al: Radiologic manifestations of sarcoidosis in various organs. *Radiographics* 24:87-104, 2004.

Cross-Reference

Thoracic Radiology: THE REQUISITES, 2nd ed, pp 188-190.

Comment

CT demonstrates numerous small nodules, located predominantly in an axial distribution, coursing along the bronchovascular bundles. This distribution of nodules is associated with a relatively limited differential diagnosis, including sarcoidosis, lymphangitic carcinomatosis, lymphoma, and Kaposi's sarcoma.

Sarcoid nodules, which represent noncaseating granulomas, are typically perilymphatic in distribution. Such nodules are predominantly located along the bronchovascular bundles, radiating from the hila in an axial distribution. Less frequently, the nodules are located in the interlobular septa and subpleural lymphatics, both peripherally and along interlobar fissures. Note that several of the nodules in this patient are located peripherally and adjacent to pleural surfaces.

A recent study demonstrated that CT images of patients with sarcoidosis frequently reveal evidence of small airways disease such as a mosaic pattern of lung attenuation and air trapping on expiratory images. It has been postulated that small airways disease in sarcoid may arise from one of two possible mechanisms: intrinsic granulomas within the small airways or extrinsic peribronchiolar fibrosis.

The combination of airways involvement and interstitial involvement in patients with sarcoidosis may result in heterogeneous patterns of functional impairment on pulmonary function tests. Patients with sarcoidosis may demonstrate a variety of pulmonary function test abnormalities, including restrictive, obstructive, and combined restrictive and obstructive patterns.

Notes

1. This patient's preoperative chest radiograph (not shown) prior to coronary artery bypass graft (CABG) surgery was normal. What is the most likely cause of the anterior mediastinal mass in this case?

2. Is this a common complication?

3. What is the most serious complication of this finding?

4. Is thrombosis a common finding in patients with venous graft aneurysms?

Saphenous Vein Graft Aneurysm Following CABG Surgery

1. Aneurysm of a saphenous vein bypass graft.

2. No.

3. Dehiscence of the anastomosis with associated life-threatening hemorrhage.

4. Yes, approximately one half of such aneurysms are partially thrombosed.

Reference

Nishimura K, Nakamura Y, Harada S, et al: Saphenous vein graft aneurysm after coronary artery bypass grafting. *Ann Thorac Cardiovasc Surg* 15:61-63, 2009.

Cross-Reference

None.

Comment

The chest radiograph shown in the first and second figures demonstrates a well-circumscribed anterior mediastinal mass located to the left of midline, in close proximity to surgical sutures related to the CABG procedure. The presence of an anterior mediastinal mass in a patient who has undergone CABG should raise the suspicion of an aneurysmal venous graft. The diagnosis can be confirmed with contrast-enhanced CT or MRI. The contrast-enhanced CT image in the third figure confirms the diagnosis of an aneurysm that contains a large amount of peripheral thrombus.

Aneurysms of saphenous vein grafts are a rare but serious complication of CABG and are typically detected 10 to 20 years after the surgery. *False aneurysms,* which are characterized by a disrupted vessel wall, are more common than *true aneurysms,* which are characterized by an intact vessel wall. False aneurysms are most commonly located at the anastomotic sites. Such aneurysms have been described in association with wound infection, intrinsic weakness of the graft wall, and iatrogenic trauma to the vein during harvesting. In contrast, true aneurysms are identified most commonly within the body of the graft. True aneurysms are thought to arise owing to progressive atherosclerosis related to exposure of saphenous vein grafts to systemic blood pressure.

Venous graft aneurysms are often asymptomatic and discovered as an incidental finding on routine chest radiographs. When symptomatic, patients generally present with symptoms of myocardial ischemia. Complications of venous graft aneurysms include myocardial infarction, distal embolization, fistula formation to the right atrium or right ventricle, and rupture and secondary hemorrhage. Treatment includes resection of the aneurysm and myocardial revascularization. Catheter-based coil embolization may be considered in high-risk surgical patients.

Notes

1. In an HIV-positive patient, are these CT findings typical of *Pneumocystis jiroveci* pneumonia?

2. What do the centrilobular branching and nodular opacities shown in the figures represent?

3. What term has been coined to describe this pattern?

4. What is the most common type of pulmonary infection to occur in HIV-positive patients—*Pneumocystis*, bacterial, or mycobacterial?

Infectious Small Airways Disease in Acquired Immunodeficiency Syndrome

1. No.

2. Impacted bronchioles.

3. Tree-in-bud.

4. Bacterial.

Reference

Aviram G, Fishman JE, Boiselle PM: Thoracic infections in human immunodeficiency virus/acquired immune deficiency syndrome. *Semin Roentgenol* 42:23-36, 2007.

Cross-Reference

Thoracic Radiology: THE REQUISITES, 2nd ed, p 323.

Comment

The HRCT images reveal numerous small, branching and nodular centrilobular opacities, consistent with bronchiolitis. There is also mild bronchial dilation and bronchial wall thickening. The findings are consistent with infectious airways disease. In recent years, infectious bronchiolitis and bronchitis have been increasingly recognized in HIV-positive patients. Interestingly, HIV-positive patients also have an increased prevalence of bronchiectasis.

Chest radiograph findings may include bronchial wall thickening and scattered small nodular opacities, the latter representing impacted bronchioles. A symmetric lower lobe predominance is often observed. Isolated small airways disease may be quite difficult to diagnose by conventional radiography because findings are often subtle and may mimic an interstitial pattern. The HRCT features of small airways disease are characteristic and include small (2- to 4-mm) centrilobular branching opacities and nodules, which represent bronchioles impacted with inflammatory secretions. The branching opacities represent bronchioles in profile (oriented in the plane of the transverse CT image), whereas the nodules represent bronchioles in cross section (oriented perpendicular to the image). The term *tree-in-bud* has been used to describe this characteristic appearance. In an HIV-positive patient, this pattern is most closely associated with a variety of infectious organisms, but it is only rarely associated with *Pneumocystis jiroveci* pneumonia.

Notes

1. This patient underwent renal transplantation 2 months ago and now presents with low-grade fever and nonproductive cough. What is the most common viral pneumonia to occur in solid organ transplant recipients?

2. Is *Pneumocystis jiroveci* pneumonia a common opportunistic infection in transplant recipients?

3. What are the characteristic microscopic features of cytomegalovirus (CMV)?

4. Has CMV pneumonia increased or decreased in prevalence among solid organ transplant recipients in the last decade?

CASE 151

CMV Pneumonia in an Organ Transplant Recipient

1. CMV.

2. No—it is rarely observed owing to widespread prophylaxis and occurs primarily in those who are non-compliant with prophylaxis regimens.

3. Cellular enlargement and intranuclear inclusion bodies.

4. Decreased.

Reference

Poghosyan T, Ackerman SJ, Ravenel JG: Infectious complications of solid organ transplantation. *Semin Roentgenol* 42:11-22, 2007.

Cross-Reference

Thoracic Radiology: THE REQUISITES, 2nd ed, pp 126-127.

Comment

Following renal transplantation, patients are at risk for a variety of infections due to the effects of immunosuppressive therapy. A knowledge of the interval between transplantation and the development of pulmonary infections can help you predict the types of organisms that are likely to cause pulmonary infections.

During the first month following transplantation, the immunosuppressive agents have not yet had a profound effect on the patient's immune system. Opportunistic infections are unusual during this period. Infections are usually caused by organisms that are typically encountered in patients with normal immunity after surgery, particularly gram-negative organisms, and commonly occur owing to aspiration or wound catheter-related infections.

Immunosuppression is usually most severe during the second to sixth months following renal transplantation. T-cell–mediated immunity is most severely depressed, placing patients at highest risk for viral and fungal infections. CMV is the most common viral agent to affect these patients, but prophylactic preventive strategies have markedly reduced the prevalence of CMV infection in the posttransplant setting. Radiographs may show a reticular or nodular pattern and, less commonly, consolidation and discrete lung nodules and masses.

After the sixth month, the immunosuppression regimen is gradually tapered. As the patient's immune system recovers, the organisms that most commonly produce pneumonia in this period are those responsible for most community-acquired pneumonias, such as *S. pneumoniae*. Because immunosuppressive agents are tapered but not discontinued, patients continue to remain at risk for opportunistic infections, particularly fungal organisms.

Notes

1. This patient has severe pulmonary artery hypertension, pulmonary edema, and a normal pulmonary venous wedge pressure. What is the most likely diagnosis for this triad of findings?

2. Is this disorder associated with a favorable prognosis?

3. In this disorder, which vessels (veins or arteries) are usually enlarged and which are of normal caliber?

4. What is the cause of venous occlusion in this disorder?

Pulmonary Venoocclusive Disease

1. Pulmonary venoocclusive disease (PVOD).

2. No.

3. Enlarged central pulmonary arteries and normal-caliber veins.

4. Intimal fibrosis.

Reference

Resten A, Maitre S, Humbert M, et al: Pulmonary hypertension: CT of the chest in pulmonary venoocclusive disease. *AJR Am J Roentgenol* 183:65-70, 2004.

Cross-Reference

Thoracic Radiology: THE REQUISITES, 2nd ed, p 328.

Comment

PVOD is a rare disorder characterized by obstruction of the pulmonary veins and venules by intimal fibrosis. Increased resistance to pulmonary venous drainage results in pulmonary artery hypertension. The classic triad associated with this condition includes severe pulmonary artery hypertension, radiographic evidence of pulmonary edema, and a normal wedge pressure. However, many affected patients do not have this triad. Affected patients typically present with symptoms of orthopnea, progressive dyspnea, fatigue, and syncope.

The etiology of this disorder is unknown, but it has been described in association with viral infection, environmental toxins, chemotherapy, radiation injury, contraceptives, and intracardiac shunts. A genetic predisposition has also been reported. There is no effective treatment for venoocclusive disease, and it is usually fatal within a few years of diagnosis. Currently, lung transplantation is the only therapy that appears to improve the prognosis of patients with this disorder.

The most commonly observed CT findings in PVOD are smoothly thickened septal lines, multifocal regions of ground-glass opacity, pleural effusions, enlarged central pulmonary arteries, pulmonary veins of normal caliber, and enlarged mediastinal lymph nodes. In the figures, note the presence of numerous thickened septal lines, multiple foci of ground-glass attenuation, slight enlargement of the segmental pulmonary arteries (increased arterial-bronchial ratio), as well as a small left pleural effusion.

Resten and colleagues compared CT findings in patients with PVOD with those with primary pulmonary arterial hypertension. They found that centrilobular ground-glass opacities, septal thickening, and mediastinal lymphadenopathy were significantly more common in patients with PVOD. Thus, the presence of these findings in a patient with pulmonary hypertension should suggest the diagnosis of PVOD. A definitive diagnosis requires lung biopsy.

Notes

1. What two conditions are most likely to present with multiple tracheal masses?

2. How can MRI help distinguish amyloid from other causes of tracheal masses?

3. This patient also had laryngeal lesions (not shown). Which diagnosis is most likely?

4. What virus is associated with this condition?

Tracheobronchial Papillomatosis

1. Papillomatosis and amyloid.

2. Amyloid demonstrates characteristic low signal intensity on both T1W and T2W sequences.

3. Papillomatosis.

4. Human papillomavirus.

Reference
Prince JS, Duhamel DR, Levin DL, et al: Nonneoplastic lesions of the tracheobronchial wall: radiologic findings with bronchoscopic correlation. *Radiographics* 22:S215-S230, 2002.

Cross-Reference
Thoracic Radiology: THE REQUISITES, 2nd ed, pp 297-299.

Comment
This patient presented with large airway obstruction. CT demonstrates multiple, cauliflower-like masses extending into the tracheal and central airway lumens. This patient also underwent laryngoscopy, which revealed several sessile laryngeal lesions. The presence of laryngeal and tracheal lesions is most suggestive of papillomatosis.

Laryngeal papillomatosis is an uncommon condition characterized by the presence of multiple squamous papillomas within the larynx. This disorder is seen primarily in children. Extension of the disease into the trachea and bronchi is referred to as *tracheobronchial papillomatosis* and occurs in approximately 5% of cases. Isolated tracheobronchial disease is seen more frequently in adults than in children. Rarely, there is dissemination into the lung parenchyma.

The radiographic and CT manifestations of papillomatosis include multiple wartlike and larger cauliflower-like growths projecting into the trachea and central airways. Larger lesions, as shown in this case, are less frequently observed. On MRI, the lesions demonstrate intermediate signal intensity, which contrasts with the characteristic low signal intensity associated with amyloidosis. When the lung parenchyma is involved, CT findings include centrilobular opacities, nodules, and cavitary nodules.

Presenting symptoms depend on the site of involvement. Laryngeal involvement frequently results in hoarseness. Tracheobronchial involvement is associated with symptoms of stridor, wheezing, hemoptysis, and recurrent infections. In children with isolated laryngeal involvement, spontaneous remission is commonly observed. With airway involvement distal to the larynx, however, spontaneous remission is less common.

Notes

1. List at least five causes of tracheal stenosis.

2. What is the difference between tracheal stenosis and tracheomalacia?

3. Is idiopathic laryngotracheal stenosis more common in men or women?

4. What is the preferred treatment for this condition?

Idiopathic Tracheal Stenosis

1. Trauma, infection, sarcoidosis, Wegener's granulomatosis, relapsing polychondritis, amyloidosis, tracheobronchopathia, osteochondroplastica, and COPD.

2. *Tracheal stenosis* refers to a fixed narrowing; in contrast, *tracheomalacia* refers to excessive collapsibility of the trachea during expiration.

3. Women.

4. Surgery (laryngotracheal resection).

Reference

Boiselle PM, Catena J, Ernst A, Lynch DA: Large airways: tracheal and bronchial stenoses. In: Boiselle PM, Lynch DA, Eds. *CT of the Airways.* Toronto, Springer, 2008, pp 130-131.

Cross-Reference

Thoracic Radiology: THE REQUISITES, 2nd ed, pp 291-292, 293.

Comment

The axial CT image in the first figure demonstrates luminal narrowing due to circumferential wall thickening of the proximal trachea. The sagittal two-dimensional reformation image in the second figure shows that the stenosis is limited to a small portion of the cervical trachea.

The patient presented in this case has idiopathic tracheal stenosis. Such patients present with narrowing of the subglottic trachea, often accompanied by laryngeal narrowing, with no history of prior intubation, trauma, infection, or systemic illness. When accompanied by laryngeal involvement, this condition is referred to as *idiopathic laryngotracheal stenosis.*

This disorder typically affects middle-aged women. Affected patients may present clinically with symptoms of shortness of breath, wheezing, stridor, and hoarseness. Although no definitive etiology has been identified, gastroesophageal reflux disease has been suggested as a potential causative factor. The diagnosis is often delayed by approximately 2 years before an accurate diagnosis is made.

The radiologic appearance of this condition is variable. The length of the stenosis may range from 2 to 4 cm in craniocaudad dimension. The affected portion of the airway is often severely narrowed to less than 5 mm in diameter. The margins of the stenotic airway may be smooth and tapered (as in this case) or irregular, lobulated, and eccentric. When tracheal stenosis presents with the latter appearance, a primary tracheal neoplasm is an important diagnostic consideration. There are a variety of surgical and nonsurgical treatment options. Surgery is the preferred treatment and is potentially curative. Palliative endobronchial treatment should be reserved for patients who are not operative candidates.

Notes

1. Are normal bronchioles usually visible on CT scan images?

2. Name the term that is used to describe nodular and linear branching centrilobular opacities due to small airways disease.

3. Is this pattern pathognomonic for TB?

4. Where in the secondary pulmonary lobule are bronchioles located?

Small Airways Disease
(Infectious Bronchiolitis)

1. No—normal bronchioles are below the resolution of CT (and HRCT).

2. Tree-in-bud.

3. No.

4. In the center of the secondary pulmonary lobule, adjacent to the pulmonary artery.

Reference

Silva CIS, Müller NL: Bronchiolitis. In: Silva CIS, Müller NL, Eds. *Imaging of the Chest.* Philadelphia, Saunders, 2008, pp 1071-1095.

Cross-Reference

Thoracic Radiology: THE REQUISITES, 2nd ed, pp 321-325.

Comment

The CT images demonstrate numerous small nodular and branching linear opacities with a centrilobular distribution. The CT appearance is characteristic of a proliferative bronchiolitis, a pattern that is frequently described as *tree-in-bud* because of its resemblance to a tree budding in springtime.

Although the tree-in-bud pattern was originally described in conjunction with TB, it is by no means pathognomonic for this process. Rather, it may be associated with a wide variety of bronchiolar diseases.

An infectious etiology is most common. Acute infectious bronchiolitis is most frequently associated with respiratory syncytial virus, adenovirus, and *Mycoplasma* pneumonia. Other important infectious etiologies include mycobacterial and fungal organisms. Other causes of proliferative bronchiolitis include aspiration and diffuse panbronchiolitis. The latter is a chronic disease of unknown etiology that occurs almost exclusively in Asians.

Chest radiographs of patients with minimal small airways disease may be normal. In patients with more extensive disease, a fine nodular pattern may be apparent, often accompanied by reticular opacities. CT is helpful in differentiating small airways disease from a true miliary pattern. The latter is characterized by a random distribution of small nodules; in contrast, small airways disease is associated with a centrilobular distribution of small nodular and branching (tree-in-bud) opacities.

Notes

1. Which portion of lung parenchyma is abnormal, the areas of increased or decreased lung attenuation?

2. What characteristic allows you to make this distinction?

3. What term is used to describe this pattern of variable lung attenuation?

4. How can you differentiate pulmonary vascular disease from small airways disease as a cause of this pattern?

Mosaic Pattern of Lung Attenuation Secondary to Small Airways Disease

1. Decreased.

2. Fewer and smaller-caliber vessels within the low-attenuation areas compared with other portions of the lung.

3. Mosaic pattern.

4. Obtain expiratory CT images—only small airways disease demonstrates air trapping.

Reference

Lynch DA: Imaging of small airways disease and chronic obstructive pulmonary disease. *Clin Chest Med* 29:165-179, 2008.

Cross-Reference

Thoracic Radiology: THE REQUISITES, 2nd ed, pp 323-324.

Comment

The CT image demonstrates a mosaic pattern of lung attenuation, with geographically marginated areas of low attenuation in both lungs. There are several possible causes for a mosaic pattern, including small airways disease, vascular disease, and infiltrative lung disease (manifesting as foci of ground-glass opacification). In the former two entities, the low-attenuation areas are abnormal. In the last entity, the foci of increased attenuation are abnormal.

When confronted with a pattern of variable lung attenuation, carefully compare the size and number of vessels between the areas of relative low and high attenuation. When the caliber and number of vessels are similar, the areas of relative increased attenuation are abnormal. This appearance is seen in a variety of entities that are characterized by the presence of ground-glass opacities, including acute interstitial infections such as *Pneumocystis jiroveci* pneumonia and chronic infiltrative lung diseases. In contrast, a reduction in size and number of vessels within the areas of low attenuation area implies that the foci of low attenuation are abnormal. Such an appearance can be seen in pulmonary vascular disorders, such as chronic pulmonary embolic disease, and small airways disease, such as obliterative (i.e., constrictive) bronchiolitis. In cases of small airways disease, the diminished vasculature occurs secondary to reflex vasoconstriction due to hypoxia. Expiratory CT can help to distinguish between vascular and small airways etiologies of mosaic attenuation. Only small airways disease is associated with air trapping on expiratory scans.

Notes

1. What unusual infection is associated with a "cyst within a cyst" as shown in the figure?

2. What term is used to describe the air collection within the cyst in the first figure?

3. What is the significance of this finding?

4. Do these cysts have a predilection for the lower lobes of the lungs?

Echinococcus Cysts

1. Echinococcus.

2. Meniscus or crescent sign.

3. It is a sign of impending cyst rupture.

4. Yes.

Reference

Martinez S, Restrepo CS, Carrillo JA, et al: Thoracic manifestations of tropical parasitic infections: a pictorial review. *Radiographics* 25:135-155, 2005.

Cross-Reference

Thoracic Radiology: THE REQUISITES, 2nd ed, pp 115, 116.

Comment

Echinococcus granulosus is the cause of most human forms of hydatid disease. It occurs in two forms: pastoral and sylvatic. The pastoral form is more common. In this form, sheep, cows, or pigs are the intermediate hosts and dogs are the definitive host. This form of infection is particularly common in the sheep-raising regions of southeastern Europe, the Middle East, Northern Africa, South America, Australia, and New Zealand.

The hydatid cyst contains three layers: the pericyst, an acellular laminated membrane, and an inner germinal layer that generates daughter cysts. The liver is the most common site for echinococcal cysts, accounting for approximately 70% of cysts. The lung is the second most common site.

On chest radiographs and CT scans of patients with *Echinococcus* cysts, you may observe single or multiple well-circumscribed spherical or oval masses. If a cyst communicates with the bronchial tree, air may enter the space between the pericyst and the laminated membrane, producing a thin crescent of air around the periphery of the cyst. In this case, the first image shows a meniscus sign, which has been reported to indicate impending cyst rupture. Note the presence of cyst rupture on the second image, which was obtained 2 weeks after the first image.

When bronchial communication occurs directly into the endocyst, expulsion of the cyst contents may produce an air-fluid level. Once the cyst has ruptured, its membrane may float on the fluid. The term *water lily sign* has been used to describe this characteristic appearance. It is important to know that these characteristic radiographic signs are rarely observed in association with this entity.

When intact, most hydatid cysts are asymptomatic. On cyst rupture, there is usually an abrupt onset of cough, expectoration, and fever. Other manifestations include pneumothorax, pleuritis, lung abscess, parasitic embolism, and anaphylaxis. Percutaneous aspiration of such cysts has generally not been considered safe owing to the possibility of inciting an allergic reaction or spreading the infection.

Notes

1. Which bronchus is more frequently ruptured, the left or the right?

2. What percentage of cases of acute tracheobronchial injury are associated with a pneumothorax?

3. Rupture of which mainstem bronchus is more commonly associated with pneumomediastinum without pneumothorax?

4. Is bronchial rupture more common than tracheal rupture?

Posttraumatic Bronchial Stricture

1. Right.

2. Approximately 70%.

3. Left mainstem bronchus, because it has a longer mediastinal (extrapleural) course.

4. Yes.

Reference

Kaewlai R, Avery LL, Asrani AV, Novelline RA: Multidetector CT of blunt thoracic trauma. *Radiographics* 28:1555-1570, 2008.

Cross-Reference

Thoracic Radiology: THE REQUISITES, 2nd ed, pp 162-164, 167.

Comment

Tracheobronchial injury is an uncommon but serious complication following blunt thoracic trauma. The mainstem bronchi are affected in approximately 80% of cases, followed by the trachea (15%) and distal bronchi (5%). Most injuries occur within 2.5 cm of the carina. Airway injury is frequently accompanied by upper rib fractures. Note the presence of healing rib fractures in this case, an important diagnostic clue to a traumatic etiology.

Imaging findings can be classified as early and late. Early findings include pneumothorax, pneumomediastinum, and subcutaneous emphysema. Pneumomediastinum without pneumothorax is most common when the mediastinal, extrapleural portion of the airway is ruptured. Pneumothoraces occur in approximately 70% of patients with an airway injury. Such pneumothoraces are typically severe and refractory to chest tube drainage.

In the setting of a complete bronchial rupture, a pneumothorax may be accompanied by the *fallen lung sign.* This sign refers to a collapsed lung that sags away from the hilum toward the diaphragm, reflecting its loss of attachment to the hilum. The lung falls inferiorly when the patient is upright and posteriorly when the patient is supine.

The diagnosis of tracheobronchial injury is often delayed. Late imaging findings are related to the development of granulation tissue and stricture within the injured bronchus, a process that occurs within 1 to 4 weeks of injury. Late imaging findings include postobstructive atelectasis, pneumonia, abscess, and empyema. The images in this case demonstrate a late presentation of bronchial rupture, manifested by complete collapse of the right lung due to granulation tissue obstructing the injured bronchus.

Notes

1. Name at least one sign of upper lobe volume loss present in this case.

2. Name at least two entities that may be associated with conglomerate masses in the upper lung zones.

3. What chronic infiltrative lung disease does chronic berylliosis most closely resemble?

4. Is chronic beryllium disease immunologically mediated?

Chronic Beryllium Disease

1. Cephalad displacement of the left hilum; left juxtaphrenic peak sign.

2. Silicosis, sarcoidosis, TB, coal worker's pneumoconiosis, and berylliosis.

3. Sarcoidosis.

4. Yes—it represents a cell-mediated hypersensitivity reaction to beryllium bound to tissue proteins.

Reference

Chong S, Lee KS, Chung MJ, et al: Pneumoconiosis: comparison of imaging and pathologic findings. *Radiographics* 26:59-77, 2006.

Cross-Reference

Thoracic Radiology: THE REQUISITES, 2nd ed, pp 213-214, 215.

Comment

Chronic beryllium disease (also called *berylliosis*) is a systemic granulomatous disorder caused by exposure to beryllium metal or its salts in the form of dust, fumes, or aerosol. The major sources of occupational exposure include the aerospace and electronics industries, the manufacturing of gyroscopes and nuclear reactors, the processing of ceramics, and the development or handling of beryllium alloys in the manufacturing of airplane landing gear, electronics, and a variety of household appliances. There is typically a latency period of 10 to 20 years between exposure and the onset of chronic berylliosis.

Chronic berylliosis is an immunologically mediated disorder that may involve multiple organ systems, including the lungs, lymph nodes, skin, liver, spleen, and bone marrow. The characteristic histologic finding is the epithelioid granuloma, which cannot be distinguished from the noncaseating granuloma of sarcoidosis.

The lungs are the most commonly involved organs, and exertional dyspnea is a frequent presenting symptom. Radiographic findings in patients with chronic berylliosis are quite similar to those observed in patients with sarcoidosis. Small nodular or reticulonodular opacities are the most common finding and may involve all three lung zones; conglomerate masses may also develop. Chronic disease may manifest as a linear pattern of pulmonary fibrosis accompanied by upper lobe volume loss, architectural distortion, and emphysematous bullae.

A history of exposure to beryllium can help differentiate this entity from sarcoidosis. Because the imaging and pathologic features are not specific, a diagnosis of chronic berylliosis can be confirmed by a patch test showing hypersensitivity to beryllium. Chronic beryllium disease is treated with steroids. Patients with symptomatic chronic berylliosis have a poor prognosis.

Notes

A

B

C

1. Name four congenital lung diseases that may manifest on CT with cystic or cystlike findings.

2. Name three possible imaging manifestations of intralobar sequestration.

3. What is the most common location of a bronchogenic cyst?

4. What is the primary characteristic of congenital lobar emphysema?

Cystic Adenomatoid Malformation (CAM)

1. Congenital lobar emphysema, cystic adenomatoid malformation (CAM), intralobar sequestration, bronchogenic cyst.

2. Solid-water density mass, area of consolidation, air-containing single or multicystic lesion.

3. Mediastinum; most often in the subcarinal region or near the central airways.

4. Progressive overdistention of a lobe secondary to an intrinsic bronchial obstruction due to a cartilage anomaly or deficiency or to compression by an extrinsic vascular structure or mass. A polyalveolar form also occurs.

Reference

Rosado-de-Christenson ML, Stocker JT: Congenital cystic adenomatoid malformation. *Radiographics* 11:865-886, 1991.

Cross-Reference

Thoracic Radiology: THE REQUISITES, 2nd ed, pp 67-68.

Comment

CAM of the lung is a rare hamartomatous lesion that represents anomalous development of lung bud elements that would have become terminal bronchioles and alveolar ducts; its cystic components communicate with the major bronchi. CAM is usually detected in the first 2 years of life but may occur in adults (10% to 20%). Affected adult patients may be asymptomatic or present with recurrent infection or hemoptysis. The imaging manifestations correlate with the three types of CAM. Type 1 manifests as unilateral single or multiple air-filled cysts; in some cases, a single dominant cyst may be surrounded by smaller cysts; type 2 manifests as multiple small uniform cysts; type 3 lesions typically manifest as a solid mass or area of consolidation. Although CAM has been considered a unilateral disease, CT has been reported to show evidence of bilateral involvement in some patients. Affected patients are at increased risk to develop bronchioloalveolar carcinoma (BAC). The definitive treatment is surgical excision. In neonates with CAM and associated severe respiratory distress, the clinical situation associated with this lesion may constitute a surgical emergency.

The original classification of CAM of the lung was recently expanded to include two additional entities that are neither cystic nor adenomatoid; this category of lesions may now be referred to as *cystic pulmonary airway malformation (CPAM)*.

Notes

1. Which six infectious diseases are recognized by the Centers for Disease Control and Prevention (CDC) as posing the greatest threat for use in bioterrorism, with highest potential for public health impact?

2. What are the characteristic chest CT findings of inhalational anthrax infection?

3. Name the vector for transmission of hantavirus.

4. How is pulmonary anthrax infection transmitted?

Inhalational Anthrax Infection

1. Anthrax, plague, smallpox, botulism, tularemia, and hemorrhagic fever.

2. Mediastinal and hilar high-attenuation lymphadenopathy and pleural effusions (both of which may enlarge rapidly over days); and peribronchovascular pulmonary edema.

3. Rodents.

4. Inhalation of anthrax spores from infected animal products (such as wool) or as a result of bioterrorism.

Reference

Frasier AA, Franks TJ, Galvin JR: Inhalational anthrax. *J Thorac Imaging* 21:252-258, 2006.

Cross-Reference

Thoracic Radiology: THE REQUISITES, 2nd ed, pp 118-119.

Comment

The threat of bioterrorism remains a reality of 21st-century life. Several infectious agents are recognized by the CDC as having the highest potential for public health impact. These diseases include inhalational anthrax, plague, smallpox botulism, tularemia, and hemorrhagic fever. Anthrax is unique in that imaging studies may allow for prompt diagnosis and institution of life-saving therapy before organ damage is irreversible. In 2001, anthrax spores were placed in envelopes and mailed through the United States Postal System.

Following inhalation, anthrax spores are transported to mediastinal lymph nodes, where they germinate for 2 to 30 days, followed by the second phase of the illness, characterized by stridor, respiratory failure, and shock. Death may occur despite antibiotic therapy.

In the early phase of the illness, the chest radiograph typically demonstrates mediastinal widening and unilateral or bilateral hilar enlargement, frequently accompanied by pleural effusions. Peribronchovascular airspace opacities occur, but parenchymal consolidation is usually not extensive. The presence of mediastinal widening and pleural effusions helps to distinguish inhalational anthrax from community-acquired pneumonia.

CT may reveal characteristic high-attenuation (hemorrhagic) mediastinal and hilar lymph nodes that may rapidly enlarge over days. Rapidly enlarging pleural effusions and peribronchovascular edema are also common CT findings. Early recognition of anthrax and prompt administration of antibiotics before the onset of fulminant illness has the potential to dramatically improve patient survival.

Notes

1. Name two diseases that may manifest as ground-glass opacity and cysts in the lungs.

2. What are the most characteristic CT findings of *Pneumocystis jiroveci* pneumonia?

3. What are the most characteristic CT findings of lymphocytic interstitial pneumonia (LIP)?

4. Name four clinical syndromes that are associated with LIP.

Lymphocytic Interstitial Pneumonia

1. *Pneumocystic jiroveci* pneumonia, LIP.

2. Bilateral perihilar or diffuse symmetric ground-glass opacity that may progress to consolidation; thin-walled cysts may occur, predominantly in the upper lobes.

3. Extensive ground-glass attenuation and scattered thin-walled cysts.

4. Sjögren's syndrome, pernicious anemia, chronic active hepatitis, myasthenia gravis, and viral infection.

Reference

Mueller-Mang C, Grosse C, Schmid K, et al: What every radiologist should know about idiopathic interstitial pneumonias. *Radiographics* 27:595-615, 2007.

Cross-Reference

Thoracic Radiology: THE REQUISITES, 2nd ed, p 192.

Comment

LIP is part of the spectrum of IIPs and is a lymphoproliferative disorder within the spectrum that ranges from follicular bronchiolitis to low-grade lymphoma. The diffuse form of this order is referred to as *LIP;* the focal form is referred to as *pseudolymphoma.* The nonneoplastic entity of LIP must be distinguished from lymphoma by immunologic stains.

Although the cause of LIP is unknown, it may be associated with abnormalities in the immune system—such as Sjögren's syndrome, pernicious anemia, chronic active hepatitis, and myasthenia gravis—or may be secondary to viral infection. It may also occur in children with AIDS.

The best imaging clue is the presence of ground-glass opacities and scattered thin-walled cysts. Other CT findings of LIP may be arrayed along the lymphatic pathways of the lung: centrilobular nodules and thickening of interlobular septa and bronchovascular bundles. Symptomatic patients may be treated with steroids and other immunosuppressive agents; some cases show spontaneous remission without treatment. The incidence of neoplastic transformation of LIP has been reported to be as high as 50% of cases.

Notes

1. Name three smoking-related interstitial lung diseases.

2. Is honeycombing a characteristic CT feature of desquamative interstitial pneumonia (DIP)?

3. What general pathologic findings in the pulmonary interstitium and the alveolar airspaces may result in ground-glass opacity on thin-section CT?

4. Which primary pulmonary malignant neoplasm most often manifests as ground-glass opacity on thin-section CT?

Desquamative Interstitial Pneumonia (DIP)

1. Langerhans' cell histiocytosis, DIP, and RB-ILD.

2. No.

3. Mild thickening of the interstitium, partial filling of the airspaces, or both in combination.

4. BAC.

Reference

Heynemann LE, Ward S, Lynch DA, et al: Respiratory bronchiolitis, respiratory bronchiolitis–associated lung disease, and desquamative interstitial pneumonia: different entities or part of the spectrum of the same process? *AJR Am J Roentgenol* 173:1617-1622, 1999.

Cross-Reference

Thoracic Radiology: THE REQUISITES, 2nd ed, p 195.

Comment

DIP is a rare interstitial pneumonia that occurs almost exclusively in cigarette smokers. Affected patients typically present with nonproductive cough and progressive dyspnea. The term "desquamative" is a misnomer; the histology of DIP was originally thought to represent desquamated pneumocytes but it is now recognized as widespread alveolar filling with macrophages containing dusty brown ("smoker's") pigment, with inflammatory infiltrates in the alveolar septa.

Although classified as an "idiopathic" interstitial pneumonia, 90% of cases of DIP are found in cigarette smokers and the disease is thought to represent part of the histopathologic spectrum of smoking-related interstitial lung diseases that also includes pulmonary Langerhans cell histiocytosis, and RB-ILD.

The chest radiograph may appear normal or demonstrate hazy ground-glass opacity in the lower lung zones. The predominant finding on HRCT is ground-glass opacity that may be patchy, diffuse, or peripheral in distribution and is typically lower zone predominant. Reticulation and honeycombing are uncommon HRCT findings. Small cystic airspaces may occur within areas of ground-glass opacity in 32% to 75% of cases. Differential diagnostic considerations include NSIP, RB-ILD, and hypersensitivity pneumonitis.

Notes

1. What are the most common indications for performance of pleurodesis?

2. What agent is used to perform PET imaging?

3. Which is more common, pleural metastases or primary pleural malignancy, such as mesothelioma?

4. What is the typical latency period between asbestos exposure and development of malignant mesothelioma?

CASE 164

Pleurodesis

1. Intractable pleural effusions, most often malignant; recurrent pneumothorax.

2. ^{18}F-fluorodeoxyglucose (FDG).

3. Metastases.

4. 30 to 40 years.

Reference

Gilman MD, Aquino SL: State-of-the-art FDG-PET imaging of lung cancer. *Semin Roentgenol* 40:143-153, 2005.

Cross-Reference

None.

Comment

PET scanning using FDG is a molecular imaging technique that is widely used to image and stage malignant tumors. Some benign pleural conditions, including empyema and thoracotomy-related pleural thickening, may show increased FDG uptake to varying degrees.

Pleurodesis is a procedure in which talc or other chemicals are introduced into the pleural space through a thoracoscopic or open surgical approach to induce inflammation, scarring, and adhesion formation between the visceral and the parietal pleural surfaces. The two leading indications for pleurodesis are treatment of large pleural effusions (benign or malignant) and recurrent pneumothorax. Pleurodesis results in pleural thickening and a chronic granulomatous reaction that is FDG-avid on PET imaging and thus may mimic pleural malignancy (i.e., metastases, mesothelioma, lymphoma).

Other benign thoracic conditions that may occasionally show increased FDG uptake include pulmonary hamartoma, lipomatous hypertrophy of the cardiac interatrial septum, and rounded atelectasis.

Notes

Note: Page numbers followed by f refer to illustrations.

Schwannoma, vs. ganglioneuroma, 68
Scintigraphy
    of ascending aortic aneurysm, 147-148
    of carcinoids, 158
    of Kaposi's sarcoma, 162
Scleroderma, interstitial lung disease secondary to, 83-84
Septic infarcts, 123-124
Sequestration
    extralobar, 276
    intralobar, 275-276
Severe acute respiratory syndrome (SARS), round pneumonia in, 66
Shingles (zoster), 170
"Signet ring" sign, in bronchiectasis, 90, 194
Silica, occupational exposure to, 82
Silicone stents, 294
Silicosis, 81-82
    complicated, 82
    simple, 82
Small airways disease
    infectious, 315-316
        in acquired immunodeficiency syndrome, 305-306
    mosaic pattern of attenuation secondary to, 317-318
    sarcoidosis and, 302
Small cell carcinoma, of lung, 108
Smokers
    cigarette
        desquamative interstitial pneumonia in, 332
        lung cancer in, 210
        pulmonary nodules in, 210
        squamous cell carcinoma in, 248
    marijuana, bullae in, 230
Solitary fibrous tumors, of pleura, 251-252
Solitary pulmonary nodule. See Pulmonary nodule(s), solitary.
Somatostatin receptors, in carcinoids, 158
"Split pleura" sign, in empyema, 72
Squamous cell carcinoma
    bronchial, mucoid impaction secondary to, 249-250
    esophageal, 44
    lung, 108
    tracheal, 248
Stenosis
    laryngotracheal, idiopathic, 314
    tracheal, 211-212
        idiopathic, 313-314
Stent, tracheal, fractured, 293-294
Sternal dehiscence, following median sternotomy, 223-224
Sternal wires, displacement of, 224
Sternoclavicular joint dislocation, 145-146
Sternotomy, median, dehiscence following, 223-224
Strangulation, associated with ruptured hemidiaphragm, 144
Stricture(s)
    bronchial, post-traumatic, 321-322
    tracheal, 150, 212
Subcarinal lymph nodes, enlarged, 79-80
Subclavian artery, right, aberrant, with aortic dissection, 273-274
Subpulmonic pleural effusion, 33-34. See also Pleural effusion.
Sulcus tumor, superior, 127-128
Superior sulcus tumor, 127-128
Superior vena cava, thrombosis of, 182
Superior vena cava syndrome, 181-182
Sweat test, abnormal, in cystic fibrosis, 56
Swyer-James syndrome, 267-268
Syphilis, ascending aortic aneurysm caused by, 148, 156
Systemic sclerosis. See Scleroderma.

T
Telangiectasia, hereditary hemorrhagic, 91-92
Tension pneumothorax, 6. See also Pneumothorax.
Thoracic aortic aneurysm, 94
Thoracic inlet mass, goiter as, 102
Thoracic lymphoma, AIDS-related, 98
Thromboembolism, pulmonary, 255-256
Thrombosed saccular aortic aneurysm, 263-264

Thrombosis, of superior vena cava, 182
Thymic carcinoma, 77-78
    vs. invasive thymoma, 78
Thymic cyst, 295-296
Thymic hyperplasia, 213-214
Thymic mass, 77-78
    differential diagnosis of, 78
Thymolipoma, 61-62
Thymoma, 78
    invasive, 78
Thyroid carcinoma, metastatic, 259-260
    extrapleural masses secondary to, 37-38
Thyroid goiter, 101-102
Toxicity
    amiodarone, 299-300
    bleomycin, 175-176
Trachea
    adenoid cystic carcinoma of, 247-248
    diverticulum of
        air cyst associated with, 221-222
        Mounier-Kuhn syndrome with, 239-240
Tracheal bronchus, 297-298
Tracheal papillomatosis, 311-312
Tracheal stenosis, 211-212
    idiopathic, 313-314
Tracheal stent, fractured, 293-294
Tracheal strictures, 150
Tracheoarterial fistula, 150
Tracheobronchial injury, blunt trauma causing, 322
Tracheobronchial involvement, by tuberculosis, 280
Tracheobronchial papillomatosis, 312
Tracheobronchomalacia, 246
    in relapsing polychondritis, 266
Tracheobronchomegaly, congenital, 239-240
Tracheoesophageal fistula, 150
Tracheomalacia, 150, 245-246
Tracheostomy tube
    abnormal angulation of, 150
    cuff of, overinflation of, 149-150
"Tram-track" sign, in bronchiectasis, 90
Transection, aortic, trauma-induced, 99-100
Transeophageal stripe, thickening of, in esophageal carcinoma, 43-44
Transplant recipient, cytomegalovirus pneumonia in, 307-308
Transplantation
    bone marrow, obliterative bronchiolitis associated with, 232
    heart, Nocardia infection following, 253-254
    kidney, CMV pneumonia following, 307-308
    lung, rejection following, 277-278
Transthoracic needle biopsy
    CT-guided, 203-204
    for bronchogenic carcinoma, 4
Transudative pleural effusion, 34. See also Pleural effusion.
Trauma. See also specific type, e.g., Fracture(s).
    aortic transection due to, 99-100
    chest, aortic injury due to, 100
    lung opacification near sites of, 28
"Tree-in-bud" lung opacities
    in small airways disease, 306, 316
    in tuberculosis, 134
Tricuspid endocarditis, septic infarcts and, 124
True aneurysm, 94, 304
Tuberculosis, 117-118
    Ghon lesion in, 86
    involving airways, 279-280
    miliary, 15-16
    post-primary, lung cavitation due to, 57-58
    Ranke complex in, 85-86
    reactivation, 133-134
Tumor(s). See specific tumor, e.g., Neurogenic tumor (ganglioneuroma).
Tumor-node-metastasis (TNM) staging, of lung cancer, 4, 108, 180

U
Uterine leiomyoma, 234